Teamworks

Transforming Health Care's Error-Prone Culture

w☉rks

Mitchell Morrison, Ph.D.

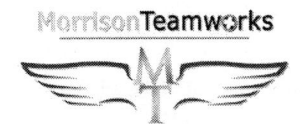

MorrisonTeamworks

www.morrisonteamworks.com

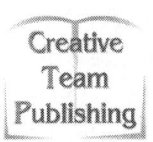

Creative Team Publishing

Creative Team Publishing
San Diego

© 2013 by Mitchell Morrison.

All rights reserved. No part of this book may be reproduced, stored in a retrieval system or transmitted in any form or by any means without the prior written permission of the publisher, except by a reviewer who may quote brief passages in a review distributed through electronic media, or printed in a newspaper, magazine or journal.

Permissions and Credits in Order of Appearance:

Mitchell A. Morrison, Doctoral Dissertation, Northcentral University, Copyright 2012.

Scripture taken from the *Holy Bible, New International Version*. (NIV), Copyright 1973, 1978, 1984 International Bible Society. Used by permission of Zondervan Bible Publishers. All rights reserved.

Definition of "communication" by Glen Aubrey in *Core Teams Work Their Principles and Practices*, © 2007 Glen Aubrey, Creative Team Publishing, is used by permission.

Mont's Ten Basic Rules for Success in Your New Management Job, Copyright 2004 by Mr. Mont Smith, is used with permission.

ISBN: 978-0-9855979-6-2
PUBLISHED BY CREATIVE TEAM PUBLISHING
www.CreativeTeamPublishing.com
San Diego
Printed in the United States of America

Cover Design by Justin Aubrey

Endorsements on behalf of *Teamworks: Transforming Health Care's Error-Prone Culture*

Aaron E. Bair

Teamworks hits the mark, giving providers an evidence-based framework to improve emergency medicine care. As we build our simulation and virtual care programs, I look forward to new advances in error mitigation as we educate residents, attendings, professors, and staff in aviation-style communications, based largely on *Teamworks: Transforming Health Care's Error-Prone Culture* and its accompanying study volume, *Teamworks Transformation Guide*.

~ Aaron E. Bair, MD, MSc Associate Professor Emergency Medicine Medical Director, Center for Health and Technology Medical Director, Center for Virtual Care, UC Davis Medical Center

Mont Smith

Brilliant work! CDR Mitch Morrison is a Coast Guard aviation leader whose passion for safety transformation is refreshing. A superb description of aviation teamwork ontology, this is essential reading for the business community, health care, the airlines, corporate, military, EMS, general aviation, and other high-risk industries. Even though I've been flying and promoting aviation safety for nearly 50 years, his book helped me to better understand underlying factors of teamwork success and failure on and off the flight deck.

~ Mont Smith, Director of Safety, Airlines for America, Washington, D.C. and former President, Coast Guard Aviation Association

Angelique Ashby

Our hospitals and medical care organizations are some of the best in America, providing cutting-edge service for over 2.5 million metropolitan area patients. Dr. Mitch Morrison's research, conducted here in Sacramento, combines the proven science and professionalism of aviation with a new and innovative perspective of communication and leadership to advance patient safety. I've known Mitch for years—he's a respected community leader and hard-working military officer who exudes humility and compassion. A great read!

~ Angelique Ashby, Vice-Mayor, City of Sacramento, CA

Spence Byrum

Dr. Mitch Morrison has nailed it in *Teamworks*! I've worked with over 600 hospitals, ASCs (Ambulatory Surgery Centers), LTACs (Long Term Acute Care facilities), and physician practices, and I absolutely believe that the greatest barrier to adopting the principles and practices Mitch describes in his book is a cultural hierarchy where autonomy is the core value. The very people who we need desperately to champion a cultural change frequently complain that the applicability of "aviation" principles to their practice is "cookbook medicine." Many claim tools such as checklists and standardized procedures detract from their autonomy and lack a personal touch. By helping us understand the key elements of human error in *Teamworks*, Dr. Morrison helps us see that these objections are not only dangerous, but absurd. Very simply put, we need to choose between an option that significantly improves patient safety by using the principles of high reliability and the old, antiquated model of care delivery that does not. From an ethical perspective, delivering care demands that we "get it right" the first time. Our *Befindlichkeit* (you'll understand shortly) needs to be that it is our moral obligation, our sacred trust, to significantly decrease the chance for human error in health care. *Teamworks* provides the template for us to do just that.

~ Spence Byrum, Managing Partner, Convergent HRS, LLC, "High Reliability Solutions for Healthcare™"

Joel Bales

Impressive work! *Teamworks* is a welcome and recommended addition to the important discussion of improving patient safety through aviation team training methods. Dr. Morrison's rigorous qualitative research systematically exposes the need for continued health care improvement emulating the success of the aviation industry during the past 30 years. He analyzes the effectiveness of current patient safety efforts and recommends process changes with potential to impact health care delivery culture through error reduction strategies. I welcome and recommend this resource to better understand and apply aviation safety principles in achieving health care's imperative to improve delivery.

~ Joel D. Bales, MA, MHA; Fellow, American College of Healthcare Executives; Project Management Professional (PMP) ®, Health Information Technology

Antonio Cortés

This book will become a game-changing resource for enhancing the reliability of modern medical processes and it also stands as a shining example of the underdeveloped field of qualitative research methods. Dr. Morrison leverages the costly lessons learned from the aviation industry's dramatic reduction in accidents over the last half century to expose concepts with potential to significantly enhance medical reliability. His thoughts are the product of thousands of cockpit hours as a naval aviator and have been refined through rigorous peer-reviewed research. It only makes sense that medicine, the most human of fields and one also heavily dependent on team leadership and followership, will benefit from actionable research associated with other high-consequence settings. Now it is up to the proactive safety leaders in the medical profession to enact the concepts—a challenge of vital importance and one in which we all share a vested interest!

~ Antonio Cortés, Ph.D.—Safety manager and reliability researcher, former Air Force and airline pilot

Timothy Reed

Commander (CDR) Morrison explains how the major transformations needed in American Health Care might be found using the principles from aviation safety culture and practice. This is needed in every aspect of health care practice to bring about the radical improvements possible—and deserved—in patient safety and outcomes. The cultural shifts for the kind of teamwork and non-defensive examination of adverse events in aviation run counter to the training of many physicians and other health care professionals. From my experience, the training and coaching necessary to bring about continuous process improvement in health care are often slow and expensive but very rewarding. The application of CDR Morrison's ideas would speed up the learning within care teams while creating an environment that encourages even faster learning, change, and organizational knowledge. Imagine—what if these ideas were applied to the "cost" of the process as well as patient safety?

~ Timothy Reed (Retired), Health Care Executive, Kaiser Permanente, Southern California Region

Gary Raff

This book comes at a critical time in our thinking about healthcare delivery in the United States. For too long health care professionals and teachers have not given enough emphasis on techniques of communication and the importance of teamwork in all aspects of medical care. How to learn to function as a team and the benefits of this approach seem like simple concepts but my experience has shown me that it is often far from simple to do. We need more books like this to highlight the importance of how to create a culture of communication, respect, continued quality improvement and improved outcomes. As a medical professional I demand it and as a patient I expect it. Shouldn't you too?

~ Dr. Gary Raff, Chief Pediatric Cardiac Surgery, Associate Professor of Surgery, University of California, Davis

Teamworks

*Transforming Health Care's
Error-Prone Culture*

works

Mitchell Morrison, Ph.D.

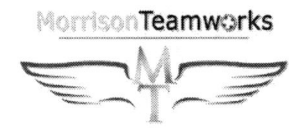

MorrisonTeamworks

www.morrisonteamworks.com

Foreword
Aviation

Captain Craig Hoskins, Vice President of Safety, JetBlue Airways

When Dr. Mitch Morrison asked me to write a Foreword to his book, I was both honored and humbled. In addition to our association for several years as Coast Guard colleagues, we also share a passion for safety. Coincidentally with Dr. Morrison's book, my interest in the parallels between the aviation and health care professions was furthered by my recent participation on a panel for the Society of Medical Decision Making, sharing aviation safety knowledge with medical leaders.

Presently we are experiencing the best commercial aviation safety record in U.S. history. This did not happen by luck or by chance. It has been the result of a combination of technological advances, automation and most importantly, the cultural shift in human performance. In aviation, technological advances took us a great distance in travel speed and mechanical reliability. This left human performance both as a risk and as an opportunity for improvement in aviation safety.

We all can agree that we are prone to making errors, no matter what the setting: aviation, nuclear power, oil production, medicine, or other endeavors. How do we reduce the frequency of these errors? And how do we mitigate the impact when errors occur? Answers to these questions for medicine could come from the cross pollination of aviation safety's best practices to health care.

Commercial aviation safety best practices in the U.S. are the result of several years of collaboration among many stakeholders. Manufacturers, airlines, and regulatory agencies have all worked together without ego or corporate boundaries. These industry efforts have also been continuous, since as the industry changes, so do the risks, requiring continuous improvements in safety initiatives.

The number of aviation safety best practices is extensive and they share very important themes. These include teamwork, communication skills, and decision making. Could these themes also be relevant in health care?

Regarding teamwork, envision a group of people that have never met, gathering at the departure gate in an airport. They have about thirty minutes to make introductions and complete the necessary pre-flight checks to prepare an aircraft for flight. This group quickly forms a team, referred to as an "Air-Crew" that will assume responsibility for numerous lives. In the world of health care, is it possible that a group of strangers could quickly form a team, who would together and assume responsibility for the lives of others?

This "teaming" occurs thousands of times per day in aviation, to transport people and in health care to conduct medical procedures. Forming effective teams that can function in a high-risk environment doesn't just happen. In aviation it has been the result of studying and learning lessons from previous accidents or incidents, or simply put: reactive improvements. But as the accident/incident rate has declined it has provided an opportunity for the aviation community to shift its focus to a proactive approach.

Being proactive is much easier said than done for it requires a culture that is willing to embrace change. Some of these changes have included enhancing communication skills, training, team-building, decision-making, policy revisions and procedure development (e.g. checklist design), plus one that is often overlooked: reporting. All have contributed to improved safety.

Another necessary and important change in human behavior is developing an investigative and blame-free culture. To enable identification of the areas of potential risk that contribute to human error an organization needs to create a culture of non-attribution and non-retribution. This is not an option. Members of an organization have to feel comfortable to report the "near misses" and leadership needs to use that data to focus on the "what" and not the "who." Identifying the "what" provides limitless opportunities for risk mitigation strategies that will:

- Keep errors from occurring when possible
- Catch the errors that couldn't be prevented
- Reduce the consequences of the errors that were not caught

Again, as U.S. commercial aviation experiences the best safety record in decades, one has to remember it was not done overnight. Looking back over thirty years to when my aviation career began, what we do now is far different from what was done then. Aside from technological advancements, the commercial aviation profession has seized the opportunity for human performance improvements and made many changes, some of which are discussed above and more of which will be described in this book. It will always be a journey for we are all human.

Conversely, how was health care administered thirty years ago? Is it the same today? Apart from equipment advances, has the human performance element in health care advanced in similar ways to that of commercial aviation? The answer to the last question is found in Mitch's book, *Teamworks: Transforming Health Care's Error-Prone Culture*. I hope you will open the next page as I did, open your mind, and enjoy the read.

~ Captain Craig Hoskins

Foreword
Health Care

Dr. James Battles
Agency for Healthcare Research and Quality

Healthcare in the United States is not safe, as pointed out in the Institute of Medicine (IOM) report *To Err is Human*, nor is it effective as pointed in the IOM's *report Crossing the Quality Chasm*. As the IOM noted more than a decade ago, healthcare lacks a culture of safety and far too many patients are harmed by a process of care that is supposed to help patients get better.

A recent report issued by the Inspector General of the U.S. Department of Health and Human Services (HHS) in 2010 noted that one in seven Medicare patients is harmed during their care. Healthcare is truly a high risk industry characterized by dangerous hazards to an individual seeking care.

John M. Eisenberg, the late director of the U.S. Agency for Healthcare Research and Quality (AHRQ) noted that healthcare is a team sport. However, when the causes of patient harm events are examined, the leading contributing factors are lack of communication and poor teamwork among healthcare professionals. These breakdowns in communication and teamwork have deadly consequences for patients. Paul M. Schyve, M.D., Senior Vice President of the Joint Commission on the Accreditation of Healthcare Organizations (The Joint Commission) has observed, "Our challenge… is not whether we will deliver care in teams, but, rather, how well we will deliver care in teams."

In *To Err is Human*, the recommendation was made that the lessons learned relative to teamwork from other high hazard industries such as aviation, nuclear power, and the military should be applied to healthcare.

The good news in healthcare is that when organizations seriously address the culture of safety and improve teamwork, patient care is dramatically improved. In

Veteran's Administration (VA) hospitals it has been shown that teamwork training has reduced surgical mortality. In the area of obstetrical care in labor and delivery the number of birth injuries and birth trauma to mothers and babies has been reduced when improved teamwork and simulation are used in combination. The reduction in birth trauma has led to a significant reduction in malpractice claims and significant cost savings.

The AHRQ and the Department of Defense (DoD) have developed a public domain curriculum and resource materials to support improvements in teamwork. The program known as TeamSTEPPS has been implemented worldwide by healthcare organizations from individual hospitals to complete hospital systems in many clinical domains. Where institutions have successfully implemented TeamSTEPPS or other teamwork improvements efforts, care has improved, a stronger culture of safety has emerged, and patients notice these improvements as indicated by an increase in patient satisfaction and patient experience of care survey results.

TeamSTEPPS and improved teamwork training have had a positive impact on the care provided to our combat troops in Iraq and Afghanistan. When TeamSTEPPS goes to war, our troops benefit, and lives are saved.

We have a long way to go in healthcare, but efforts at applying the lessons learned from aviation and other high hazard industries in improving teamwork are making a difference. The more we learn about approaches to improve teamwork and apply that new knowledge, the safer healthcare will become.

A major component of healthcare reform and a reduction in the rising cost of healthcare will be focusing on teamwork and the culture of safety. Effective teamwork saves lives and lowers the cost of healthcare.
~ James B. Battles, Ph.D., Social Science Analyst, U.S. Agency for Healthcare Research and Quality, Adjunct Professor of Bioinformatics, Uniformed Services University of the Health Sciences, and Captain, United States Navy (Retired)

Dedication

Dedicated to those who have suffered loss through tragedy.
We remember. Not to blame, but to learn.
In doing so, we change who we become and
transform our future.

"...To act justly and to love mercy and
to walk humbly with your God."
~ Micah 6:8 (NIV)

w⊛rks

Welcome to *works*. We invite you to join us on a worthwhile journey about life-transformation. Discovery occurs when the disciplines of science, innovation, and communication come together to improve any personal or professional environment.

In *Teamworks: Transforming Health Care's Error-Prone Culture*, Dr. Mitch Morrison illustrates one example of how *works*, works. He illustrates aviation's team-oriented behaviors for error mitigation, and then within a historicity context presents research observations regarding health care's transformation. The journey of discovering, learning, and applying effective methods of error mitigation in aviation becomes a model for reducing errors in health care. What works in one application, works in another.

Dr. Morrison introduces us to a common theme on this journey. It is one he calls, your *Befindlichkeit*. (It's pronounced *Beh-FINNED-leh-kite*.) The term, based on the philosophy of Martin Heidegger, really means "a moment of discovery." It's that instance of welcome realization often termed *the Aha moment*. *Befindlichkeit* happens when knowledge, understanding, and application of truth are shown to change lives for the better—fulfilling a worthwhile goal for all who appreciate personal growth and process improvement.

This entire process of discovery, or *Befindlichkeit*, centers around a core question. Vast and untapped frontiers of knowledge and understanding await. Take flight and answer the question for yourself:

> **How would a richer understanding of *being* influence what you *know* to transform what you *do*?**

The bigger picture in asking and answering this question is not just the knowledge of a matter; rather, through the science of ontology, it is the understanding of why and how matters influence organizational culture. Embedded strategies include systems theory, root cause analysis, and double-loop learning.

Future research and writing revolve around a central and recurring theme: simply put, <u>these ideas *work*</u>. For example, teamwork works, organizational structure works, ontology works, collaboration works, and decision-making within an environment of mutual respect and cooperation works. You get the idea.

In an environment where desires for personal and professional growth are shared and understood, three core imperatives become the interlocking values in both personal and organizational intention. The *Befindlichkeit* of learning and applying them in one area becomes the springboard of learning and applying them in another. These tenets compose the essence of living and working cooperatively on the journey of fulfilling greater causes and providing positive and sustainable improvements.

Inspiring Distinction

Serving People

Building Community

All three imperatives cooperate with one another. In fact, each one intersects with the other two. Quantifiable results emerge from these values when they are activated, and committed people engage with one another to see them come to fruition.

Now is the time for a new journey of unbounded discovery, changing and improving behaviors with a goal of benefitting everyone. When a better understanding of being intersects with knowledge and application, positive outcomes result. *This* is what *works* is all about.

Together, we have the freedom and the encouragement to discover how *works* works! We simply have to start.

**Are you ready? If so, then let your journey begin!
It's your move.**

works

www.wxrks.com

A Two-Book Set

Teamworks

Transforming Health Care's

Error-Prone Culture

and

Teamworks

Transformation Guide

Teamworks and the *Teamworks Transformation Guide* compose a two-part set. The study guide follows the chapter format of the book, and is suited for seminars, coaching, or individual reflection.

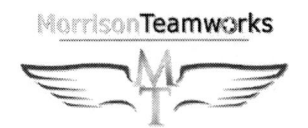

works

MorrisonTeamworks

Table of Contents

Foreword
  Aviation
    Captain Craig Hoskins, Vice President of Safety,
      JetBlue Airways 13

Foreword
  Health Care
    Dr. James Battles, Agency for Health Care
      Research and Quality 19

Dedication 23

wxrks 25

A Two-Book Set 31

Introduction
  Safety Culture Transformation 43
    Crew Resource Management (CRM) 47
    Checklists 48
    Briefings 48
    Reporting-Analysis 48

Behavioral Change	51
Shared Understanding	52

Chapter One

Is Medicine a Team Sport?	57
A **Teamworks** Culture	64
Unhealthy Autonomy and Hierarchy	67
Teamworks Core Values	68

Chapter Two

A Clearing in the Woods	69
Befindlichkeit: Where Do We Find Ourselves Now?	69
Aviation Teamwork Heuristic	72
Husserlian and Heideggerian Phenomenology	73
Epistemology and Ontology	74
Disclaimer	75
What Is Your *Befindlichkeit*?	75
Lived Experiences	79
Two Central Research Questions	86

A Transformation from Military to Civilian Life

    The Jim Crismon Letter   89

Chapter Three

  A New and Useful Tool   95

    Population of Interest   97

    Specific Population   100

    Participant Selection Process   101

    Number of Participants   102

    Participant Demographics   103

    Table 1: Demographic Profile Findings   104

    Materials and Instruments for the Study   107

    Triangulation   108

    Credibility   109

    Exploration   111

    Description   115

    Interpretation   120

    Methodological Assumptions,

        Limitations, and Delimitations   122

    Assumptions   122

    Limitations   126

Delimitations	131
Ethical Assurances	132
Protection from Harm	132
Informed Consent	133
Right to Privacy	134
Honesty with Professional Colleagues	135

Chapter Four

Root Cause Perspective: More than Mere Problem Solving	137
One for the Birds	137
Chernobyl	140
Catholic Healthcare Partners	142
Root Cause Analysis	143
Challenger Disaster	145
A Learning Culture	151
A Learning Culture and Accountability	152

Chapter Five

Aviation Safety Transformation: Roots of Change	155

Roots of Aviation Safety Transformation 158

Birth of the Federal Aviation
    Administration (FAA) 160

Eastern 401 162

Tenerife 164

Portland 165

Chapter Six

Aviation Teamwork: Translating Key Tools to
Health Care Settings 171

    Aviation Teamwork Heuristic 179

    Double Loop Learning 179

    Crew Resource Management (CRM) 181

    Checklists 197

    Briefings 201

    Reporting-Analysis 205

Chapter Seven

Bridging Aviation Teamwork: From Theories to
Field Research 215

    Moments of Discovery 217

Seeking "Aha" Moments	222
The Impetus for Organizational Transformation	224
Inspiring Distinction, Serving Others, and Building Community: Values Forming the Vision of **Teamworks**	224

Chapter Eight

Real-Life Excerpts from Health Care Providers	227
Data Statistics and Distillation Steps	229
Learning from the Data	230
First Segment: How Do Health Care Personnel Describe Their Experiences with Learning Aviation Teamwork Methods?	232
Implicit Learning	232
Real-time Learning	241
Second Segment: How Do Health Care Personnel Describe Their Experiences Applying Aviation Teamwork Methods in Health Care Settings to Mitigate Root Causes of Medical Errors?	246

Structure	246
Influence of Egos	251
Third Segment: Bonus Themes	254
Transformation	254
Teamwork	260
Leadership	269
Fourth Segment: Vivid Real-Life	
Error Accounts	276

Chapter Nine

Now What?	289
Tension of Autonomy, Hierarchy, and Blame	293
Evaluation of Findings	298
Comparison with Other Studies	302
Effects upon Field of Study	305
The Wildcard of Generational Differences	309
Mont's Ten Basic Rules for Success in Your New Management Job	310
Learning from Past Mistakes	315
Summary	317

Chapter Ten

    A Call to Arms   319

        Enter **Teamworks**   320

        A New Theory and Its New Behaviors   327

        Teamworks Recommendations   329

        Recommendations for Practice   330

        Mutual Learning and Living   331

        Recommendations for Future Research   333

        Alignment and Application   335

Twelve O'clock High   339

Acknowledgements   343

About the Author   345

Glossary—Definitions   347

Index   357

References   367

Appendix A

    Phenomenological Interview Guide   395

Appendix B

    Respondent Recruiting Letter   401

Appendix C

    Informed Consent Form   403

Appendix D

    Schematics   407

        Figure D1: Data Collection   407

        Figure D2: Exploration   408

        Figure D3: Descriptive Analysis   409

        Figure D4: Interpretive Analysis   410

Introduction

Safety Culture Transformation

Safety culture transformation in the United States health care system is a strategic imperative to mitigate medical errors. I don't think health care practitioners and leaders intend to perpetuate an error-prone culture; however, a puzzling dynamic remains. Health care continues educating the best and brightest to become independent and autonomous, a flawed hierarchical model which I think has been self-replicating, something to expect rather than fix. Too many errors have resulted in unnecessary injuries and even worse, the tragedy of lost lives. For those concerned with improving health care quality, a new understanding and a set of changed behaviors is an immediate task.

In the breakthrough Institute of Medicine (IOM) study *To Err is Human* published in 1999, researchers suggested healthcare improvements, in part, could be achieved through adaptation of aviation-based safety methods. Let's face it: once airborne, there is no forgiveness regarding preparations of the aircraft or crew prior to flight for a successful takeoff, cruise, approach and landing. Aviation has taken giant leaps forward in addressing and mitigating loss before it happens. And many of these lessons have come from bitter experience and a desire to prevent further loss.

Simply put, the question is: "Can health care learn from aviation's experience and knowledge?" In short, the answer is a resounding "yes!"

My interest and passion for understanding safety culture transformation stems from my own experience as an aviator and safety practitioner. Over 30 years in my military and civilian pilot career I have observed many teamwork iterations both on and off the flight deck.

Teamwork works not because teams' practices are static; in fact, they change constantly. They have to. What does not change are the desires of people to improve according to the lasting principles of cooperation, leadership, and encouragement. These principles frame the foundation for a healthy environment with effective leadership and education. These principles must be taught, learned, embraced, and actively employed.

This book is an adapted version of my doctoral dissertation research study that I defended in April 2012. As I researched and studied these matters in an academic setting, I came to a "clearing in the woods" to realize changes in aviation over my own career offer clear lessons for similar transformation in health care, as other authors have.

My dissertation research began in 2009, and was designed to use a qualitative method and phenomenological design to answer two core questions. The first one was: How do health care personnel describe their experiences with learning aviation teamwork methods? To address it, I explored how health care personnel describe their experiences with learning aviation teamwork methods. I found that learning aspects of health care teamwork include implicit learning styles and real-time learning for relevance; however, pedagogy lacks deliberate focus, leading to management and staff frustration. Generally, health care providers receive no formal training in the principles of cooperation, leadership, and encouragement. Often this leads to lost opportunities for improvement, efficiency, and failed efforts to resolve personnel frustration.

The second question was this: How do health care personnel describe their experiences applying aviation teamwork methods in health care settings to mitigate root causes of medical errors? I found that disclosure initiatives yielded transparency and fostered increased community accountability. Where the tough stuff (challenges) resided, however, were in the lingering traditions of autonomy and hierarchy-influenced ego-driven behavior. In short, these behaviors presented opportunities for medical errors. Unfortunately, those errors occurred, resulting in profound results for both patients and caregivers.

Aviation uses methods that I think could work within health care. Some are already in use, but their implementation is ad hoc, lacking deliberate focus. The methods I have in mind are crew resource management, checklists, briefings, and reporting-analysis. These are time-tested, recognized methods to teach, learn, embrace and employ.

Crew Resource Management (CRM)

CRM was born during the hierarchical, error-prone 1970s in aviation, when crews communicated poorly with each other and allowed minor technical distractions to create disaster. In the current generation, CRM programs remain part of the fabric in which crews train and operate.

Checklists

Checklists are a memory aid for repeated steps where humans make errors. A simple tool, checklists work very well; however, tradition, autonomy, and ego prevent more widespread use.

Briefings

Briefings keep teams on the same page in operational settings. A simple introduction, including one's name and role can make the difference between trust and exclusion in the heat of battle, whether on a flight deck or in surgery.

Reporting-Analysis

Reporting-Analysis is a systems-based process of reporting and analysis by staff, to highlight hazards, errors, and near-misses. It helps leaders navigate their progress toward organizational safety and process improvement.

My research shows that the health care community is on a clear path of change. However, health care's transformation remains marked by struggle, conflict and division across disciplines and communities that want to move toward an outlook of hope, improvement and safety. The statistics and facts you will read support this.

Conversely, health care teamwork reflects an essence of expert groups working together in a committed sense of trust and community with effectiveness and cohesion. I have found and firmly believe that most practitioners want to work better in team settings, but find themselves stuck in a culture of ego-driven tradition. They take matters into their own hands to make change, and are often successful. However, to influence lasting change, a grass roots approach isn't enough.

From my research I have learned, and will demonstrate, that health care professionals desire to learn and apply innovative teamwork for error mitigation. I will also show that community research perspectives remain divided between anecdote and evidence, and that this gap must be bridged. We need ready-to-use techniques for leaders and staff now. Solutions I will present stem from my own doctoral dissertation research with practicing physicians, nurses, and managers. I was impressed by their drive, commitment, and professionalism and sensed their anticipation of a transformation in the health care safety culture, a culture that embraces teamwork, collaboration, and continuous quality improvement.

I am convinced that great teachers must remain eager students and that effective leaders never stop being stellar followers. Health care education must emphasize transforming health care delivery, similar to study of disease and biology in medical schools and pharmacological and therapy research in laboratories.

Indeed, the medical profession knows what to do, even how to do it. I want to address the reasons behind what we do and reasons for adopting new methods. In other words, I want to address the motives behind why we should stop doing some behaviors and start doing others.

Behavioral Change

Behavioral change stems from alterations in attitude. Willful behavioral change is always superior to that which is forced. Buy-in from the health care community is critical.

Do we want to address an error-prone culture to make it better? If we do, then we must recognize the factors that inhibit the goal of error mitigation and continuous quality improvement.

First and foremost is the cultural context of learning and applying teamwork methods. These efforts take time to influence change, mitigate entrenched factors, and build consensus.

Another dynamic is the growing challenge of interpersonal communication between workers of varied ages, otherwise known as generational differences. Ethnic cultural factors may influence how teamwork is manifested.

And lastly, although we don't like to admit it when addressing safety programs, financial constraints and limited resources often limit transformation. Improving teamwork is like getting more exercise and eating healthy; we can all do better.

Shared Understanding

I see a future where lessons learned in health care can assist to transform aviation's next generation; lessons learned will transcend across communities in a continuum of shared understanding. Shared understanding is key. An environment of sharing is one of collaboration, cooperation and open communication where no one cares who gets the credit and no one dwells upon fixing blame. This is an atmosphere where all stakeholders recognize the issues and seek to support each other towards common goals as problems are addressed and solved.

The goal of this book is to save lives, to decrease injuries, and to reduce costs in health care, aviation, and other settings where teamwork is paramount. If committed people learn and take that learning to the core of their being, if actions are taken to reduce errors and help avoid preventable accidents, I as the author and you as the reader will have accomplished worthy goals. We should congratulate each other on our successes because we, too, could someday share in the benefits.

I chose the title of this book to address this truth head-on. Every good-hearted person desires a strong return for an investment of life and experience where the welfare of another is concerned. This is true in health care, aviation, and any industry where other's lives are at stake. Instead of concluding that medical errors are simply part of the culture of health care, I decided that we should do something positive to mitigate and solve this conundrum.

I am passionate about my desires to see health care improved, because I do care. If you care, too, read on. This book is for us all.

What is needed if not required for the health care industry is to transform how to teach and model behaviors that have already been proven to work in aviation. My research yielded this profound truth: Medical scholars and key stakeholders lack alignment regarding the basic teaching approach to achieve a culture of health care safety (Leape et al., 2009; Wachter, 2010). I think a small change in educational and training foundations for health care providers would foster a huge culture change and make our health system safer and more efficient. This is the goal.

We must learn from the past and present to improve the future. When viewed in the context of a historical continuum, health care's safety culture and the aviation community's development of teamwork methods represent interpretive frameworks to characterize a dynamic process of ongoing transformation, learning, and adaptation across communities.

I think aviation teamwork methods offer an opportunity to improve safety in any high-stakes pursuit. These are venues where people collaborate, cooperate and communicate effectively to accomplish a goal. This mutual interdependence is where the value of teamwork is manifest.

Explore my work and let's learn together. Join me in a spiral of shared understanding about these matters.

Mitchell Morrison, Ph.D.

Chapter One

Is Medicine a Team Sport?

At the conclusion of a bombing mission over Nazi Germany, a maintenance crewmember was amazed when an aircraft returned to base with flak holes in its wings and fuel tanks. Upon further investigation, the mechanic removed several unexploded shells. All of the unexploded shells were empty except for one. The one shell had a folded piece of paper with a note written in the Czech language: "this is all we can do for you right now" ("Small Deeds Count," 2007). A distinguished choice by one person had a profound impact for others. These laborers received no accolade or fanfare, yet lived in small community to overcome despair and join the fight in their own small way. An unknown group of heroes exercised selfless courage and fortitude to produce inert ammunition, a noble act that saved 10 American airmen.

Consider the impact of this discovery as the mechanic told the story to his superiors! What gratitude the men who flew the plane must have felt! Ten families had a husband, father, son, brother still alive to pursue their own legacy.

Early in Franklin Delano Roosevelt's Presidency, on the heels of worldwide economic depression, the gritty leader said, "The only thing to fear is fear itself." Small steps to defeat fear were "all we can do for you right now." Small steps are often the initial ones taken in any life-giving and enduring enterprise.

I believe health care systems must be transformed. Specifically, I'm convinced that health care's safety culture, if changed, could result in lives saved, unnecessary injuries prevented, and costs avoided.

If this work helps only one person avoid tragedy, it's a just undertaking. I am convinced it's worth the endeavor.

So as health care's safety culture transforms, health care community leaders must recognize the profound impact of each small step toward error mitigation. One at a time, saving the life of a child, mother, father, baby, friend, or stranger remains a worthy effort.

There are winners and losers in sports. Regarding delivery of health care, however, both caregivers and patients can be winners. How can we transform medicine into a team sport?

Look at these facts. In 1999, the Institute of Medicine (IOM) released a breakthrough study titled *To Err is Human*, which declared at least 44,000 people die in U.S. hospitals each year because of medical errors (Kohn et al., 1999). Authors of the IOM study despaired over lost patient trust and diminished health care workers' satisfaction, labeled medical errors as an epidemic, and proposed a 50%

reduction in errors (Kohn et al., 1999). Kohn et al. (1999) prescribed a national-level focus upon organizational health care process improvements, including adaptation of aviation-based safety methods (Kohn et al., 1999; Lessard, 2008; Musson & Helmreich, 2004). A decade later, patient safety ratings have advanced at an annual average of only one percent (Berwick & O'Kane, 2008; Encinosa & Hellinger, 2008; Leape et al., 2009; Wachter, 2010).

When confronted with statistics and facts like these it causes me to seek the core, the root of the problem. Here's what I found: steep hierarchies and obsolete education practices contribute to a culture of blame and fear in many health care organizations and inhibit discussion of and learning from errors (Baker et al., 2006; Leape et al., 2009; Walton, 2006).

The U.S. health system spends almost three times more per capita than Britain; however, in 2006, 89% of British doctors used electronic medical records, compared to 28% in the United States (The Commonwealth Fund, 2008). The

U.S. infant mortality rate (6.8%) is double that of Japan (2.8%) and Finland (3.3%), with the lowest states exceeding 10% (The Commonwealth Fund, 2008). Since 2000, annual U.S. health insurance administration costs have risen to almost $150 billion, an increase of 78% and 7.5% of total expenses compared to 1.9% in Finland and 2.3% in Japan (The Commonwealth Fund, 2008).

Statistics on efficiencies help us to frame the magnitude and complexity of problems that people in the U.S. health care system must contend with. Errors extend beyond patient care.

Ask yourself as I have asked within me, "If we know that errors exist and we know that they can be corrected, and that steep hierarchies, obsolete education practices, and a 'culture of blame and fear' is what stands in our way, why *shouldn't* we change that culture?"

Three decades ago, the aviation community developed teamwork methods to mitigate poor communication (Weiner et al., 1993). Musson and Helmreich (2004) suggested aviation's safety culture transformed from 1979 to 2004 as a result of teamwork methods implemented early in pilot training. Some health organizations have explored aviation teamwork methods to mitigate medical errors (Meyers, 2006; Pratt et al., 2007).

All well and good. But what do we *do* with this information? In confronting a stodgy, error-prone system, I have to agree with this: health care staff must transfer aviation teamwork methods with careful adaptation and contextual alignment (Armitage, 2009; Salas, Wilson, Burke, & Wightman, 2006).

Salas et al. (2006) recognized that health care quality could improve through use of aviation teamwork methods, but cautioned the changes would require a considerable amount of time. Leape et al. (2009) called for physician training reforms to enable transformational changes. The key for cultural change is revamping pedagogical views (Argyris, 2002; Baker et al., 2006, Conklin, 2007; Thomas,

2006). Several scholars noted that minimal data exist regarding use of aviation teamwork methods for clinical outcomes (Baker et al., 2006; Lyndon, 2008; Pratt et al., 2007).

I say we take the time, refine the methods and earnestly work for transformational change. Do you agree?

December 2009 was the ten-year anniversary of the seminal Institute of Medicine (IOM) study *To Err is Human*. Two leading patient safety scholars marked the IOM study in recent literature reviews. An original board member for the IOM study, Leape et al. (2009) declared a culture of process flaws and noted physicians are not educated to work together in teams. Wachter (2010), a prominent author of two textbooks on medical errors, asserted a lack of consensus between academics, regulators, and accreditors in the latest literature. Wachter (2010) also noted an alarming industry trend that advocates punishment for physicians who commit errors and financial penalties for the organizations in which they practice.

A Teamworks Culture

A **Teamworks** culture is all about processing flaws and finding solutions in an atmosphere of cooperation. This will include but not be limited to building consensus and reducing punishment for people who commit errors. We'll never deny the need to find the crux of the problem, but it does no good to live there and hurt the people who are trying to help. Let's design ways to help them!

Enter aviation safety practices. During the early 1990s, medical researchers became intrigued by aviation-based safety methods and explored their use in the operating room. Dr. Gaba from Stanford University and Dr. Gerhart-Schaefer in Switzerland are among the first physicians documented in literature to employ aviation methods in operating room simulation training (Helmreich, Wilhelm, Klinect, & Merritt, 2001; Musson & Helmreich, 2004; Weiner et al., 1993).

University of Texas researchers Sexton, Thomas, and Helmreich (2000), used a cross sectional survey and assessed responses to stress and teamwork of 1000+ health care personnel and 7500 pilots. A key measure reported was that 98% of pilots agreed juniors should question decisions made by seniors, which validated a well-founded culture of safety in aviation.

One cannot observe this positive result without comparing it to health care in this focus. Further research showed how health care staff assertiveness lacked similar focus (Sexton et al., 2000). Only 55% of surgeons and 25% of surgical nurses believed it appropriate to speak up when a bad decision was being made in the health care setting (Sexton et al., 2000). The anesthesia community revealed the lowest tendency to question decisions: 39% of anesthesiologists and 28% of anesthesia nurses (Sexton et al., 2000). Only one resident anesthesiologist among 10 was willing to raise concerns when errors were made. Musson and Helmreich (2004) reported lack of assertiveness of medical personnel as a contributing factor to error situations.

What if we created in health care an environment where free expression was encouraged in light of a poor decision being contemplated? What if we asked those who worked in health care to raise their concerns when they could see errors being made or about to be made?

In 1999, in *To Err is Human,* the IOM sparked significant health care community introspection of potential remedial strategies (Kohn et al., 1999). Included in the Kohn et al. (1999) study was a recommendation for further research of aviation-based methods for medical error mitigation (Musson & Helmreich, 2004). It appeared to be about time.

This kind of transformation may not happen quickly. A lot of changes have to occur, not the least of which are refreshed perceptions and attitudes that precede more effective practices. I believe health care's safety culture is transforming at a sluggish pace due to an overriding tension among key leaders. A lack of alignment in health care remains regarding how to resolve traditions of autonomy and hierarchy.

Unhealthy Autonomy and Hierarchy

At the core, unhealthy autonomy is acting on your own without seeking another's counsel "because I've always done it this way." Hierarchy that promotes isolationism is nothing more than taking and then reinforcing a closed-off shelter, hiding in a system of title and tenure without the benefit of the positive influence of others.

If we want to improve, then systems to mitigate risk must include outcomes from a culture-based transformation targeting autonomy, hierarchical traditions, and time pressures. Leape et al. (2009) released a Harvard study identifying five concepts for transforming health care: "Transparency, care integration, patient/consumer engagement, restoration of joy and meaning in work, and medical education reform" (p. 425). Ironically, the closing statement of this candid report on the status of health care's transformation was that "medical schools are producing square pegs for our care system's round holes" (Leape et al., 2009, p. 427).

If that's the case, then the pegs and the holes have to be reformed. Let's consider how.

Teamworks Core Values

Teamworks is not just the knowledge of a matter; rather, through the science of ontology, it promotes an understanding of why and how matters influence organizational culture. Embedded strategies include systems theory, root cause analysis, and double-loop learning.

Core values of **Teamworks** include:
- Inspiring Distinction
- Serving People
- Building Community

Teamworks' vision is to transform safety culture through science, innovation, and communication. Indeed, medicine *is* a team sport.

Chapter Two

A Clearing in the Woods

Befindlichkeit: **Where Do We Find Ourselves Now?**

German philosopher Martin Heidegger used the term *Befindlichkeit* to describe moments of stark encounter. Loosely translated, it means, *where do we find ourselves now?* If you will join me in shared discovery, I'll explain the theoretical context of my research perspective. The foundational aspects of the views we take while considering aviation teamwork will be helpful as we engage in the sense-making process to understand the matters at hand.

When viewed in a historical context, the aviation community's development of teamwork methods and health care's safety culture represent interpretive frameworks characterizing the dynamic process of community (e.g., health care or aviation) transformation, learning, and adaptation. These frameworks, while different from one another, represent opportunities for learning new methods and using them to effect positive change in any environment.

The transformative nature of teamwork culture applied in aviation institutional foundations is a key element of the hypothesis to improve safety in health care. I believe this because I have seen the evidence that it works.

Years of aviation safety training and experience have instilled in me a deep sense of systems-based inquiry. I considered it essential to drill into the notion of transformation, looking deep inside the how and why behind changing safety culture.

As I studied various research styles, colleagues warned me to prepare for a lot of work if I pursued qualitative methods. In retrospect, I wholeheartedly confirm their admonition. I knew that I didn't want to simply confirm a hypothesis through impersonal surveys or questionnaires, especially in another community like health care.

I wanted to experience things for myself.

Aligned with a goal of personally seeing the evidence, I considered various theoretical approaches in the realm of qualitative methods, including case study, grounded theory, and phenomenology. While I find the case study method of presenting aviation mishaps useful for learning as a practitioner, the essential elements and mechanics of this particular method as a research design didn't resonate with me. If you want to know more about case study research, consult Robert Yin's text (Yin, 2003).

Aviation Teamwork Heuristic

I studied qualitative research approaches and found grounded theory an objective design to achieve theory generation. I ran with the approach and generated a theory that I called *aviation teamwork heuristic* to contextually frame aviation's safety culture transformation. The term "heuristic" reflects a rule of thumb or frame of reference.

As a methodological design, I can confirm that grounded theory certainly met the academic requirements for rigor in methods and theory development. To complete my in-depth study of qualitative methods, I compared grounded theory with phenomenology. Canadian scholar Max van Manen extolled the strength of phenomenology to study transformation and "reach into the depth of our being prompting a new becoming." (Van Manen, 2007, p. 26).

I examined the works of two key forefathers of phenomenology whose approaches warranted further consideration: Edmund Husserl and Martin Heidegger. Their philosophical roots met with divergent focuses.

Husserlian and Heideggerian Phenomenology

Husserlian phenomenology is descriptive (eidetic) and adopts more of an empirical focus upon respondents (Flood, 2010; Patton, 2002). Heideggerian phenomenology is interpretative (hermeneutic) and includes historicity and forestructures of understanding (Conroy, 2008). Van Manen suggested the practice of phenomenology in itself served to "mediate the epistemology of Husserl and ontology of Heidegger" (p. 18).

As I contemplated the differences between epistemology and ontology, I found my own 'eureka' or 'aha' moment. Think of it as a clearing in the woods, a *Befindlichkeit*.

Epistemology and Ontology

I want to briefly explain the terms epistemology and ontology. Epistemology is a term to describe theory of knowledge. Ontology simply means a matter of existing or being. As we embark on our philosophical journey, consider what comes first: knowing or being? How would a richer understanding of *being* influence what you *know* to change what you *do*?

> How would a richer understanding of *being* influence what you *know* to change what you *do*?

The notion of ontological science captured the essence of how I viewed aviation's culture transformation and how health care could adapt a similar approach to affect patient safety. This introspective approach led me to my own *Befindlichkeit*.

But, before moving further, let's pause for a disclaimer.

Disclaimer

If you don't agree with my view, that's okay. My job is to give you a picture of what I see to build mutual understanding. You decide for yourself what you think about it. An essential factor of ontology is for you to become introspective.

What Is Your *Befindlichkeit*?

In the context of teamwork, whether in health care, aviation or other venues, look inside to the depth of your being. How was it formed and produced?

In short, what is your *Befindlichkeit*?

My research revealed that qualitative methods were well suited to understand respondents in their work settings and preferred over other designs for accomplishing detailed research into systems processes (Conklin, 2007; Morrow, 2005). In development of the methods I would use for conducting my research and study, I noted a lack of qualitative data regarding the impact of aviation teamwork methods on health care's safety culture.

As I reviewed the literature to explore health care's safety culture transformation, I found that several scholars described root causes of medical errors stemming from steep hierarchies and obsolete educational practices (Sutker, 2008; Walton, 2006). Early on, I saw old and immovable people structures, as well as failures to embrace new ideas and innovation. These composed major stumbling blocks to process development.

Further, many scholarly works carried a tone of perplexity and frustration over a lack of health care community alignment for didactic educational philosophies (Baker et al., 2006; Campbell et al., 2007; Clark, 2008; Kliger, Blegen, Gootee, & O'Neil, 2009; Kuzel et al., 2004; Leape et al., 2009; Lewis & Tully, 2009; Lyndon, 2008; MacNulty & Kennedy, 2008; Sukkari, Sasich, Tuttle, Abu-Baker, & Howell, 2008; Sutker, 2008; Wachter, 2009; Walton, 2006). As these trends were discovered, phenomenology emerged as an apt design to elucidate the problem. We had to see the issues in order to recognize and fix them.

As I conducted my research and began writing my dissertation, the lack of consensus among health care advocates jumped out at me. My interest was particularly sparked by the lack of mandated oversight influence in health care by The Joint Commission and the Agency for Healthcare Research and Quality (AHRQ) as compared to the Federal Aviation Administration (FAA) and National Transportation Safety Board (NTSB). As I continued collecting, critiquing, and synthesizing data in writing my dissertation, I struggled with whether to present aviation teamwork in a broad or narrow context.

Cognizance of the desired contextual research framework was important in development of the core research questions. I drew charts and diagrams capturing differences between specifically applied aspects of CRM in operating rooms compared with other aspects such as checklists, briefings, and reporting used in a broader context to enhance performance in team settings. I decided to approach the study in a broader context.

Kaptchuk (2003) praised the value of a "good science to embody tension between empiricism of concrete data and rationalization of deeply held convictions" (p. 1453). I wanted to describe what it is like for someone in health care to learn teamwork, use it, and experience errors. Therefore, I could better understand the *Befindlichkeit* of why their transformation was so slow.

I didn't just want to prove that errors were happening; we all know that to be true. I wanted to discern how and why they happened, and further, to discern the how and why of the perceived inherent tension behind error mitigation strategies.

Lived Experiences

My conclusion was this: empirical, epistemological, or descriptive study of medical errors is not enough to transform health care's safety culture. Research also had to extend to the ontology of practitioners' lived experiences to understand learning and application of error mitigation tools, including aviation teamwork methods. The rubber meets the road where education validates real life experience and improvements are accomplished.

Heidegger's philosophy noted researchers should grasp contextual aspects of a phenomenon in order to deepen understanding. Events can't be studied apart from their environment.

To generate increased understanding of health care's safety culture transformation, I arrived upon a design of interpretive phenomenology (IP) with hermeneutical underpinnings. In short, I planned to collect data among health care respondents, then explore, describe and interpret the data through a lens of aviation teamwork methods.

> The rubber meets the road where education validates real life experience and improvements are accomplished.

Phenomenological methods align with root cause and systems philosophy, both of which are embedded in safety culture transformation. Larkin et al. (2006) stated IP is particularly useful in applied contexts across sciences (e.g., humanities or medicine) or communities (e.g., aviation or health care).

When viewing the context of a respondent's experience, IP allows researchers to generate deep insights and understand embedded meanings (Bradbury-Jones, Irvine, & Sambrook, 2010; Clarke, 2009). Hermeneutic research includes entry into and immersion within the hermeneutic circle, also viewed as a continuum of shared understanding between the researcher, respondents, and community at large (Smith & Osborn, 2008).

As the study concluded, I wrote a summary of findings and conclusions, and delivered an oral defense for my committee. My chair and mentors on the university committee encouraged me to contribute to the body of literature. Thus, this book.

As a basis of entry into the hermeneutic circle of the study, shared contextual historicity (Conroy, 2008) included health care community awareness of the ubiquity of error in Kohn et al.'s (1999) report and an ongoing health care safety culture transformation (Leape et al., 2009). Causes of error in one arena were seen to be causes of error in another.

A benchmark aviation framework is the 1979 NASA CRM workshop to initiate pilot culture change. Contextual "forestructures of understanding" (Conroy, 2008, p. 39) included discovery of various teamwork methods in aviation to transform aviation's safety culture (Musson & Helmreich, 2004) and learning and application of aviation teamwork methods in health care (Meyers, 2006; Pratt et al., 2007). Creswell (2003) advocated a theoretical lens as an interpretive-critical technique of data analysis. My study execution included interpretation through these contextual frameworks. Again, where teamwork methods worked in aviation, I explored a myriad of ways where they could work in health care.

The hermeneutic or interpretive circle also included a pilot study (Kezar, 2000). Before commencing the formal study, a preliminary pilot study took place with two respondents, and confirmed the value of the interview guide in capturing information related to the research problem and answering the central research questions. Conroy (2008) asserted a perspective of partnering between researcher and respondents to engender mutual exploration of emergent themes and suggested the hermeneutic circle was not a circle but a spiral in commentary development.

During the interviews, I as the researcher gave particular attention to each respondent, to elicit their true perspective of teamwork. Instead of a circular inquiry into their lived experience, I started out with simple terms, then continued in a spiral with depth and detail to capture each person's *Befindlichkeit*.

The intended approach for the study included exploration, description, and interpretation. I will explain design execution a little later.

The benefit of exploring culture transformation is increased learning among the community of researchers. Coupled with description and interpretation of findings, true knowledge can be obtained—and when embraced can evoke dramatic and positive change.

Smith and Osborn (2008) noted the iterative, flexible nature of interpretative phenomenological analysis (IPA) and asserted lack of a specific manner to execute IPA. The research process included IPA elements; however, the synthesized design in the completed study is phrased as IP.

Over the past generation, aviation's safety culture transformed, in part, through implementation of four core team-oriented concepts:

1. Crew Resource Management (CRM)
2. Checklists
3. Briefings
4. Reporting-analysis

The teamwork methods used in aviation provided a theoretical framework and basis for exploration, description, and interpretation in health care settings for increased understanding of these methods.

Research questions were intended to yield a detailed description of the lived experiences of learning and application of aviation teamwork methods by health care respondents. A unique advantage to phenomenological techniques utilized in the present study allowed constructivist exploration into the lived situations of health care experts to uncover and cluster individual lessons into a discourse of rich, meaningful understanding. And rich and meaningful understandings compose the starting blocks in a race to achieve positive change.

As I said earlier, I wanted to see for myself what health care respondents had to say about their vivid lived experiences with teamwork methods to mitigate errors. I designed the study to achieve this, and generated a rich body of data.

Interpretative phenomenology advocates broad, open questions with minimal interviewer prompts. Smith and Osborn (2008) suggested a general question to begin the interview, with more specific questions used as a funnel as necessary to explore specific areas. Morrow (2005) proposed fewer questions to generate depth and richness. In other words, methods of questioning were designed to promote truthful answers, not rote responses, and to elicit more in-depth information as an interview progressed.

Two Central Research Questions

Therefore, interviews commenced with the first of two central research questions:

> Q1: How do health care personnel describe their experiences with *learning* aviation teamwork methods?

After the respondent provided a detailed explanation of their learning experience with aviation teamwork methods, the interview moved to the second of two central research questions:

> Q2: How do health care personnel describe their experiences *applying* aviation teamwork methods in health care settings to mitigate root causes of medical errors?

Appendix A contains a detailed interview question list for the semi-structured interview. Please see p. 395.

When the respondent interaction addressed both central research questions, a more detailed interview question guide was used to explore emergent themes, clarify technical terms, and probe areas noted during data collection. The interview concluded after the respondent asked participants to comment on perceived key interview highlights.

Medical scholars do not agree on the best didactic approach to achieve a culture of health care safety (Leape et al., 2009; Wachter, 2010). But note these statistics: a dynamic process of shared responsibility, community learning, adaptation, and transformation contributed to a 74% reduction in U.S. airline mishaps from 1987 to 2006 (NTSB, 2007). From these facts we should frame a discussion of the elements of aviation teamwork methods in a health care culture transformation context. What would a reduction of over 70% of errors mean in health care and the effectiveness anyone would want where lives can be saved?

Kottke et al. (2008) noted frustrations among health care stakeholders and suggested that additional research of implementation strategies would benefit and improve health care delivery. Conklin (2007) supported the benefits of phenomenological research to improve organizational leadership and behavior. Kensella, Park, Applagyei, Chang, & Chow (2008) noted the suitability of phenomenology for understanding the lived experiences of practicing health care professionals. Phenomenology is compatible with understanding health care's safety culture transformation (Colaizzi, 1978; Groenewald, 2004; Moustakas, 1994; Patton, 2002; Shank, 2006; Trochim & Donnelly, 2008; van Manen, 2007).

Here's the bottom line: a rich body of qualitative data was collected to supplement current research into health care's use of aviation teamwork methods for error mitigation and safety culture transformation. The resulting study is worthy of our consideration.

Before presenting more details about the people involved in the study, let's look at why the timing of organizational transformation may be important.

Teamworks

A Transformation from Military to Civilian Life
The Jim Crismon Letter

As I recently contemplated career goals, I met with one of my most esteemed life mentors, 89-year-old Jim Crismon. Jim told me a fascinating story about his transition from the military to civilian life after having served in the U.S. Navy for 22 years, retiring with the rank of Master Chief Petty Officer, the senior most enlisted rank. Jim is a combat veteran of both World War II and Korea. I respect him highly. I asked Jim to write his story down. Please reflect upon it carefully:

> *Hi Commander:*
>
> *Congratulations on your move to DC and assignment as Chief, Coast Guard Aviation Safety, also your personal attainment of your PhD. You are perfectly positioned for the CAPT selection.*
>
> *I never considered the incident of breaking down the racial barriers in the Randolph County Memorial hospital in Pocahontas, Arkansas, (the*

County Seat of Randolph County where I was raised) sufficiently important enough to write it down. I had just accepted the job as Administrator of the hospital immediately after retiring from the Navy and preparing the hospital for Medicare funds was just part of the job.

It was 1966 and Medicare had recently been enacted. When I went to the hospital it was still segregated but had received notice that there was to be an inspection by the Arkansas Board of Health to determine if the hospital qualified to receive Medicare funds. There were still segregated waiting rooms, rest rooms, drinking fountains and patient rooms with "White Only" and "Black Only" signs posted. I ordered the signs taken down and advised the staff that the hospital was totally integrated.

I was making rounds of the hospital with the chief nurse and we came to a screened in porch that contained 3 or 4 hospital beds. It was June and HOT and the porch was not air-conditioned, yet there was one patient, a black man, out there. I asked the nurse if we had a room in the air-conditioned portion of the hospital where we could put the patient. She informed me that all rooms were occupied, so I asked if there was a two or three bed bedroom with a vacant bed. She said there was one vacant bed in a two-bed room but that the President of the Board of Directors of the Hospital occupied the other bed.

I pondered the situation and decided it was my job to integrate the hospital so might as well start now. I ordered the black man patient to be put in the empty bed in the room with the President of the Board. The nurse was stunned but she complied. I anticipated that my first day on the job would be my last one but never heard a word from anyone about "the integration." We passed the Medicare inspection and started receiving Medicare funds. There was never any opposition from anyone, nor any agency to the total integration of the hospital.

I hope this little memory will help you. Feel free to edit as you think it may fit.

Your Friend,

HMCM James L. Crismon, USN Ret (E-9).

Jim's story hits home for a lot of reasons. Among them:

In 1966, Arkansas was in the midst of a nationwide movement to break down racial barriers. It was no longer if it would happen; it was only a matter of when. It was the right thing to do, but some didn't agree.

Although he was simply trying to make his hospital eligible for Medicare payments, Jim's work was ground breaking, transformational in nature. He took courage in giving an order in taking down signs and that the hospital was no longer segregated.

When he ordered the nurse to house a black patient in the same room as a white patient, who happened to be the president of the board of directors, Jim displayed courage and foresight. His decision literally stunned the nurse.

Jim's decision is similar to the foresight required to spark safety culture transformation today for improved teamwork. These decisions may stun some who remain stuck in stale hierarchy, tradition and autonomy. Strong leaders must decide whether they want to transform toward safety, and if so, they must look ahead boldly.

In the latter part of 2012, health care providers were told they must post their quality scores on the internet in order to receive Medicare funds. As Jim worked to transform a country hospital in Arkansas almost half a century ago, how might an increased knowledge of teamwork ontology improve quality scores in your organization?

> Strong leaders must decide whether they want to transform toward safety, and if so, they must look ahead boldly.

More importantly, have you yet discovered your own *Befindlichkeit*?

Let's explore more.

Chapter Three

A New and Useful Tool

Put this visual in your mind. A fifteenth century king was preparing for battle when a small group of colonels approached him, looking to use some new technologies. A shrewd salesman offered machine guns, grenades, and explosives to combat their overwhelming opponents; both sides were armed only with swords and spears. The salesman hinted further of available tanks, artillery and aircraft.

Yet, the busy king wasn't interested, saying, "I haven't time for your crazy salesman; I've a battle to fight."

What new and useful tool is available to assist in fighting your next battle?

The specific problem that was addressed in my dissertation was a lack of understanding regarding learning and application of aviation teamwork methods in health care settings to mitigate root causes of medical errors. The purpose of this qualitative study was to use phenomenology to explore, describe, and interpret health care respondent experiences with learning and application of aviation teamwork methods to mitigate root causes of medical errors.

A rich body of data from fieldwork with health care experts serves to illuminate palpable contexts and critical uses of aviation teamwork methods in health care. Again, the phenomenon explored was learning and application of aviation teamwork methods in health care settings to mitigate root causes of medical errors.

Population of Interest

The specific population of interest was physicians, nurses, anesthesiologists, residents, or patient safety managers who have experienced use of aviation teamwork methods in their health care careers. Their analysis of those methods in their areas of expertise was revealing.

Interpretative phenomenological methods affirmed by Clarke (2009), Conroy (2008), Moustakas (1994), and Smith and Osborn (2008) suggest researchers champion smaller, purposeful sample sizes with more depth and detail. Therefore, a group of 10 purposively selected respondents served as the sample, with further conventions detailed later.

So who were the people involved in the process? Participants came from and fieldwork took place at various Northern California health care organizations.

Utilization of the research questions was intended to yield a detailed description of the lived experiences of health care respondents while learning and applying aviation teamwork methods. Lived experiences must include learning and application if they are truly to be lived. In short, learning becomes living with behavioral change.

So let's review: the nature of the qualitative study was exploration, description, and interpretation of health care's learning and application of aviation teamwork methods to influence safety culture transformation. The phenomenon explored was learning and application of aviation teamwork methods in health care settings to mitigate root causes of medical errors. Smith and Osborn (2008) noted interpretive phenomenology studies emphasize depth over breadth. This study included interviews with a purposively selected group of 10 respondents from Northern California health organizations, including physicians, nurses, anesthesiologists, residents, and patient safety managers.

To qualify for the study, respondents were willing to discuss their experience with aviation teamwork methods learned and applied in health care contexts to mitigate root causes of medical errors. For purposes of the study, aviation teamwork methods include Crew Resource Management (CRM), checklists, briefings, and reporting-analysis. Research took place during scheduled 60-90-minute semi-structured, one-on-one, audio-taped interviews at quiet, pre-determined private locations. Interviews were transcribed verbatim to a Microsoft Word document.

Phenomenological exploration and description steps proceeded using a combination of Smith and Osborn's (2008) and Colaizzi's (1978) methods of respondent data extraction and clustering. These synthesized methods were combined with Groenewald's (2004) method of data explication as outlined by Shank (2006). Interpretation followed a combination of hermeneutical methods advocated by Clarke (2009), Conroy (2008), Patton (2002), Shank (2006) and Smith and Osborn (2008). Following transcription of the audio-taped interview and application of the aforementioned process, a debriefing occurred in person or by telephone to confirm mutually emergent themes and enhance the study's credibility.

Specific Population

The specific population was made up of physicians, nurses, anesthesiologists, residents, or patient safety managers who had experienced use of aviation teamwork methods in his or her health care career. The estimated number of people who would qualify for the study at each location was 50-100. The sample makeup was a result of stratification through health care positions, including four physicians (three males and one female), two nurses (one female and one male) and four managers (one male and three females). Stratification occurs when a researcher has enough of a particular sample attribute and looks for balance with other attributes.

All participants reported experience at other institutions and contributed those perspective comments during interviews. Two of the managers contributed extensive nursing experience to the sample; one manager was a previous community college dean of nursing.

Participant Selection Process

Among participants, a variety of positions, experience, and organizations was sought to stratify the sample. An initial inquiry (Appendix B, p. 401) was sent via e-mail to the aforementioned Northern California health care organizations requesting purposive respondents. Following Institutional Review Board (IRB) approval in the respective institution, applicants were solicited via electronic mail. Those participants who responded to the interview query did so voluntarily.

Based on response and follow up to the solicitation in Appendix B, a preliminary telephone conversation took place to identify health care personnel willing and able to articulate their own experiences (Conklin, 2007). It was easy to identify available respondents but difficult to align schedules. Participants identified for selection but not interviewed (due to schedule conflicts or other reasons) remained in reserve until a sufficient quantity of data were collected.

Number of Participants

The minimum number of participants advocated for phenomenological studies is three (Giorgi, 2008; Thomas & Pollio, 2004). Smith and Osborn (2008) noted IP studies advocate more depth with fewer respondents and suggested beginning researchers should consider a sample size of three.

To determine a convention for the number of participants in the proposed, doctoral level qualitative study, 10 papers publishing the results of phenomenological studies over the past five years were reviewed. These 10 studies contained a low of five participants and a high of 25 participants. The low and high numbers were discarded, and analysis of the remaining eight studies resulted in an average of 8.5 respondents.

Participant Demographics

Interviews with 10 respondents occurred during the study, forming a sample of an equal number of males (50%) and females (50%). The sample contains respondents of various age groups, experience levels, national backgrounds and ethnicity.

Participants came from two organizations representative of the population of at least seven major health care institutions located in Northern California. Refer to Table 1 which follows for participant demographics.

Table 1: Demographic Profile Findings

Respondent	Position	Sex	Age[a]	Race
A	Physician	Male	35-49	Caucasian
B	Physician	Female	35-49	Caucasian
C	Nurse	Male	50+	Caucasian
D	Manager (Nurse experience)	Female	35-49	Caucasian
E	Nurse	Female	35-49	Caucasian
F	Physician	Male	21-35	Caucasian
G	Manager	Male	35-49	African American
H	Physician	Male	35-49	Caucasian
I	Manager (Nurse experience)	Female	50+	Caucasian
J	Manager	Female	35-49	Caucasian

Note: [a]The age column aggregates respondents in generational groups, i.e. Baby Boomer (50+), Generation X (35-49) and Millennial (21-35). Generational group categories adapted from "Managing the Millennials," by C. Espinoza, M. Ukleja, and C. Rusch, 2010.

The benchmark for phenomenological study completion is known as saturation (Colaizzi, 1978; Moustakas, 1996). Smedley (2007) required seven participants for saturation in a study of Australian nursing students. Kalman, Wells, and Gavan (2009) interviewed 11 Canadian nurses working on a higher degree to achieve saturation.

With the constructivist nature of phenomenology, the exact number of required participants in the study was unknown. However, 10 qualified, purposively selected respondents provided a benchmark for methodological approval to engage into research, and a group of 10 purposively selected respondents from the specific population served as the sample. The data were carefully reviewed to assess saturation, and I determined that 10 respondents were adequate to achieve study goals.

Sites of inquiry included Northern California health organizations: University of California (UC) Davis Medical Center, Sutter Health, Mercy Hospital, Kaiser-Permanente, Veterans Affairs (VA) Northern California Health Care

System, David Grant Medical Center at Travis Air Force Base, and UC San Francisco. Each site was approached, with one immediate positive organizational response.

Another positive organizational response resulted after six telephone calls, including contact with the hospital chief of staff's office. Three negative organizational responses were received after four phone calls, and two organizations failed to respond to multiple telephone and electronic mail inquiries.

Prior to commencing each interview all 10 participants signed an informed consent form (Appendix C, p. 403). Each interview took place in a private, quiet office or conference room. No payment or compensation was made for study participation.

Of those interviews scheduled, all but one took place, which was cancelled due to a respondent scheduling conflict. Another two respondents remained in reserve and were not interviewed.

Materials and Instruments for the Study

Materials and instruments for the study included an interview guide, an e-mail template to solicit respondents, and an informed consent form. During fieldwork, a more detailed interview question guide (Appendix A, p. 395) was used to explore emergent themes, clarify technical terms, and probe areas noted during data collection.

Fleming and Wentzell (2008) created a qualitative safety culture assessment tool, an instrument that influenced development of the questions and inquiry dimensions in Appendix A. Before commencing the formal study, a preliminary pilot study took place with two respondents to confirm the value of the interview guide in capturing information related to the research problem and answering the central research questions. Appendix A required no adaptation based on the results of the pilot study. During the course of the 10 interviews, no changes or additions were made to the core research questions, which were pursued to completion with all respondents. The interview guide was used to review emergent areas prior to concluding each interview.

A letter and e-mail template (Appendix B, p. 401) were used to establish contact with and identify respondents in the health care community for research. During data handling, confidentiality and anonymity of respondents followed Department of Health and Human Services protocols.

Triangulation

Data collection, processing, and analysis in the study included implementation of the phenomenological steps of exploration, description, and interpretation. A synthesis of several phenomenological designs from recent scholarly literature was executed to achieve methodology and design triangulation.

I felt it important to make sure my own use of phenomenology reflected a high degree of academic rigor while being true to my own goals and specific vision. I achieved method triangulation through studying academic examples and other scholars' work, and used the conceptual models to frame my own design.

Sampling from various organizations took place for respondent triangulation. Trochim and Donnelly (2008) equated internal validity in qualitative studies with credibility. Credibility was essential because the data gathered from respondents must remain believable.

Credibility

Credibility was maintained in the study through careful adherence to the proposed design, which had been vetted through a rigorous academic review involving several doctoral-level mentors. Morrow (2005) introduced use of a statement describing one's research perspective to increase quality and trustworthiness in qualitative research. My perspective is constructivist and systems-oriented. Frequent journaling for personal and professional reflection continued to maintain reflexivity during the study.

I'll devote more text later to describe the details of a systems perspective, but I will say this here: my own leadership philosophy is simple. It is do the right thing, care for people, and keep ego in check.

As a career military pilot with near 20 years of specialized safety education, training, and experience, I found it both exhausting and exhilarating to experience the ups and downs of going through a doctoral-level program while continuing to serve on active duty. Of course, Coast Guard core values of honor, respect, and devotion to duty influence my perspective. Cognizance of systems-based process design, such as root cause analysis and double loop learning influence my own constructivist underpinnings.

To summarize my research goals: I enjoy looking for opportunities through lessons learned, often gleaned through truthful reporting and insightful analysis. In my view, it remains important to instill trust to achieve transparency and thereby spark culture transformation.

Now let's continue with the nuts and bolts of how I conducted the study.

Exploration

Exploration and description steps proceeded using a combination of Smith and Osborn's (2008) and Colaizzi's (1978) methods of respondent data extraction and clustering. These synthesized approaches were combined with Groenewald's (2004) method of data explication as outlined by Shank (2006).

Interpretation followed a combination of hermeneutical methods advocated by Clarke (2009), Conroy (2008), Patton (2002), Shank (2006), and Smith and Osborn (2008). All transcripts, tables, and a summary of journal entries during fieldwork were retained in a separate secure file.

Pseudonyms were used for respondents to maintain confidentiality.

Confidentiality was vital because of Department of Health and Human Services protocols, academic standards, and professional dignity. I treated confidentiality with utmost importance so all respondents' identifications would remain unidentified. Explicit permission was obtained from each respondent to include their answers and our conclusions that include their answers, in this book.

The timeline for data collection for this study was from July 2011 to December 2011. Fieldwork took place during scheduled 60-90 minute interviews with respondents in their working environment or in a neutral location. Interviews transpired using a semi-structured open-ended format (Zikmund, 2003). Permission was obtained to record interviews in their entirety with a digital recording device, and field notes were taken during data collection sessions.

Respondents were given freedom to talk openly about health care's safety culture transformation despite perceived relevance to the questions. To enhance credibility, participants were encouraged to think out loud (Lyndon, 2008). Reflexivity and self-journaling were used throughout the interview process to correlate responses to the theoretical lens and identify areas of substantive significance without adding bias or leading respondents (Moustakas, 1994; Patton, 2002).

Review of the data collected in fieldwork commenced immediately following respondent interviews, in the form of descriptive and reflective field notes. To preserve the rich data collected, all interviews were transcribed verbatim into a Microsoft Word document prior to analysis.

Smith and Osborn (2008) noted the transcription time for 60 minutes of taped interview is approximately five to eight hours. A clean unedited transcript of each interview was preserved in an electronic file. The exploration phase included initial review of the transcript and field notes, and notes were made on one margin (Smith & Osborn, 2008). To increase credibility, the process included the respondents' own words (MacQueen, McLellan, Kay, & Milstein, 1998).

The first three steps of Colaizzi's (1978) method of thematic clustering and the first step of Groenewald's (2004) explication method were implemented during the exploration phase. Groenewald's (2004) first step includes bracketing, described as phenomenological reduction. Bracketing is reduction of bias and researcher influence to increase the truth and quality of respondent data (Groenewald, 2004; Shank, 2006).

Smith and Osborn (2008) suggested interviewers use as minimal prompting as possible to receive the richest data possible. I used more prompting during my first couple of interviews, and discerned quickly that transcribing and analyzing my own words were not necessarily the goal. I wanted to generate richness and thickness by hearing detailed insights from respondents. As interviews continued, I learned how to elicit thick data with minimal prompting.

A second review took place during the preliminary work, which included summarizing and paraphrasing with notes on the other margin to generate themes. A table of chronological themes was produced through repeated analysis of each individual transcript. Key narratives were marked for potential quotes in the body of the dissertation manuscript. This description covers the exploration phase, and the manuscript continued to the description phase of the phenomenological design.

Description

Continued analysis of the transcripts and tables of themes included a transition from chronological to theoretical themes. Groenewald (2004) described data explication as more compatible with phenomenology than mere analysis. Groenewald's (2004) and Colaizzi's (1978) data analysis methods were synthesized in the description phase.

Groenewald (2004) introduced a five-step method of data handling identified as explication:
1. Bracketing and phenomenological reduction.
2. Delineating units of meaning.
3. Clustering of units of meaning to form themes.
4. Summarizing each interview, validating it, and where necessary, modifying it.
5. Extracting general and unique themes from all the interviews and making a composite summary.

Colaizzi's (1978) method of thematic clustering includes the following steps:
1. Read the participant descriptions.
2. Extract significant statements.
3. Formulate meanings.
4. Organize the meanings into thematic clusters in two steps:
    a. Review the original themes and protocols.

b. Tolerate ambiguity or discrepancies between original and new themes.
5. Integrate results into an exhaustive description of the phenomenon under study.
6. Create an unequivocal statement of the structure identification.
7. Validate the structure identification through sharing with participants.

Colaizzi's remaining steps (4-7) and the first four steps of Groenewald's methods took place in the exploration phase. Each interview transcript and chronological table was reviewed and themes were clustered into a theoretical table.

Units of meaning were reviewed for literal content and compared with observations from field notes regarding non-verbal cues or voice fluctuations. This rigorous process continued into an examination to elicit principles combining insights regarding respondent data. Strauss and Corbin (1998) asserted that scholars may draw upon their own experiences during analysis.

Conroy (2008) noted the hermeneutical process seeks a confirmation of study footprints through respondent interaction. When finishing my review and analysis of each respondent interaction, I agreed with the notion of using respondents as a first reviewer to confirm the truth and purity of the data.

Therefore, following transcription of the audio-taped interview and creation of chronological and theoretical tables, a debriefing was conducted in person or by telephone to ensure respondent alignment, confirm mutually emergent themes and enhance the study's credibility and dependability (Bradbury-Jones, Irvine, & Sambrook, 2010). Creation of the theoretical table led into the interpretation phase.

As the description phase neared its conclusion, I slowly migrated from an insider (emic) to outsider (etic) perspective (Clarke, 2009). Becoming even more objective was required to achieve the interpretive aspects of using thematic clusters as a contextual lens.

I downloaded a mind-mapping program to my computer. Mind-mapping was a useful processing tool to handle the vast amounts of textual data, and I recommend it highly for those engaged in qualitative research.

Think of mind-mapping as a way to create diagrams or digital sticky notes then group them together in patterns that make sense. You can take snapshots of your digital work and extract it to a file for printing, briefing, or other purposes.

Mind-mapping allowed digital handling, grouping, and categorization of the 330 significant statements, and comparison and thematic synthesis across respondent disciplines and positions. Production of a concise mind-map summary for each respondent yielded intuitive data representations used to discern meanings, elicit themes, and write the findings and implications herein.

Interpretation

The goal of interpretation was to transition toward a double hermeneutic of the researcher making sense of the respondents' sense-making efforts during their interview (Clarke, 2009; Larkin et al., 2006; Smith & Osborn, 2008). A double hermeneutic results as the respondent works through sense-making efforts for himself or herself and the researcher determines how their experience fits in a thematic context. Then, the two discuss the process and glean deeper insights. I think you will see this in a practical way when I present my data findings.

As the interpretation phase began, I listened to the audio tapes again to re-immerse myself into each respondent's world (Conroy, 2008). Each transcript's chronological and theoretical table was reviewed and a superordinate synthesis created to transcend all respondents. Groenewald's (2004) fifth explication step was used to integrate with theoretical frameworks. The interpretation phase also transcended into imaginative aspects of description (Conklin, 2007;

Moustakas, 1994). As I engaged in this step, I tried to imagine how these attributes fit, using my researcher identity and the aviation contextual lens.

Authentic interpretation of a rich body of qualitative data through the aforementioned hermeneutic framework was executed to generate new understanding of learning and application of aviation teamwork methods in health care settings to mitigate root causes of medical errors. This was the goal.

As thematic clusters for the composite data description emerged, to increase thickness, vivid individual quotes from transcript narratives were selected for use in the dissertation manuscript (Scannell-Desch & Doherty, 2010). As outlined in Conroy (2008), interpretation considered Heidegger's three existential modes: "Authentic (own up to), inauthentic (disown), and undifferentiated (fail to take a stand)" (p. 57). It was interesting to note that all respondents affirmed their own position authentically.

As interpretation neared completion, a rich synthesis of all respondents' theoretical tables resulted in a concise list of clustered themes (Smith & Osborn, 2008). This rigorous process led to creation of an expansive interpretative narrative (Smith & Osborn, 2008). The resulting interpretative narrative was intermixed with vivid quotes and related to the literature to generate a rich body of data for increased understanding into health care's safety culture transformation.

Methodological Assumptions, Limitations, and Delimitations

Assumptions

Bias was a known limitation for the study. In the phenomenological study, the study design was followed to maintain a bias-free perspective and to collect data reflecting truth from within respondents. In an effort to mitigate bias, I documented written answers to the proposed questions prior to commencing fieldwork. (See Appendix A, p. 395.)

Wall, Glenn, Mitchinson, and Poole (2004) described an in-depth process of reflective journaling to achieve the listening characteristics during interviews to yield deep and critical respondent thinking. An honest and ethical perspective remained during journaling.

While not difficult, sometimes I didn't have profound or monumental thoughts as I reflected upon the data. The value of journaling came as I was working on my findings and conclusions.

Given my journal, I had a record of my own sense-making experience to compare, contrast and confirm thematic and contextual observations. Some people may consider journaling as a waste of time. I believe that I could not have finished the study without exercising this tool. If nothing else, journaling gives me an opportunity to empty my mind so I can move ahead with my work.

The participant selection process was a dependability threat mitigated by proactive liaison with health organization managers. I was careful to promote and maintain a dialogue with a few key contacts because we needed to establish and maintain communication to diligently schedule our meetings. So we created a liaison through electronic mail and cell phone texting. As schedule milestones emerged, we worked through the details of scheduling, meeting and debriefing.

In a 2005 safety culture study at the VA, researchers required contact with more than 90 hospitals to obtain 30 potential samples (Rosen et al., 2008). Difficulty in obtaining a commitment to engage in fieldwork was anticipated as a limitation. Further, Rosen et al. (2008) found a weakness when sampling "purely on a first come-first served basis" (p. 281). Therefore, Rosen et al. (2008) advocated use of stratified data samples of diverse participants. Inclusion of participants from different organizational cultures is aligned with Fleming and Wentzell's (2008) continuum, ranging from pathological to generative cultures. These efforts served to delimit selection bias and achieve stratification.

I am convinced that stratification was vital to the success of my study. Here's why: if I were to only sample one position in health care, i.e. nurses, then the data would not reflect a rich and broad portrayal of a given organizational culture. Therefore, in addition to nurses, I included physicians and managers. Further, I expanded the study to multiple organizations.

Assumptions regarding the population included availability to discuss learning and application of aviation teamwork methods in health care settings to mitigate root causes of medical errors. Additional assumptions included a shared understanding of interpretative frameworks, accurately represented job title, experience, and organizational affiliation, and a proper environment for data collection.

To mitigate concerns of disclosure or fears of negative information shared at respondents' environments, interviews took place at a quiet, confidential site, with emphasis on data security. Transparent information interchange occurred during fieldwork and during follow-up meetings with respondents to verify the results and establish credibility (Trochim & Donnelly, 2008).

Limitations

Credibility was not adversely impacted by poor engagement with respondents due to misunderstood questions. Open and full respondent engagement and mutual understanding remained, despite my status as a professional aviator and not a representative of the medical community.

I recognized early on that my status and inquiry techniques may conflict with one another. Therefore, I built relationships with key contacts to improve my credibility. As the study continued, these contacts advised me on how to successfully execute my work.

Morrow (2005) noted the importance of proper training for credibility in one's field when beginning a qualitative research project. I completed four years of doctoral coursework in business administration, including extensive research methods preparation and an elective healthcare administration course. To further mitigate concerns over credibility, the design included a pilot test during which no potential weaknesses were found prior to commencing the formal study. In addition, a preliminary telephone conversation took place with all respondents to build rapport and increase credibility.

Building rapport had its challenges and victories. For example, I connected with one organization with people willing and ready to conduct research. However, the protocols and procedures for approval demanded that I remain flexible with time delays and frustrations over the approval.

To ensure alignment, participants were encouraged to think out loud (Lyndon, 2008). Results of the interviews were shared with the participants to confirm mutual understanding and further decrease credibility threats. In other words, to assure that what was heard was what was said, I shared both the verbatim transcript and my detailed and excerpted mind-maps with each respondent.

Another threat to credibility was inconsistent researcher perspectives during the exploration, description, and interpretation phases. To preserve consistency and mitigate this threat, journaling and reflexivity took place (Golafshani, 2003; Groenewald, 2004; Patton, 2002). In addition, peer debriefing with a colleague allowed me to remain objective through the exploration, description, and interpretation phases.

I thought it would be more difficult to execute the data analysis. Having a sound research plan and following the plan made it possible to analyze the data. I created a detailed mind-map to outline my strategy and followed it precisely. This map is included in Appendix D, pp. 407-410.

For dependability, reflective and descriptive field notes were kept of learned experiences with a rich account of theories, contexts, and generalizations (Groenewald, 2004; Strauss & Corbin, 1998; Trochim & Donnelly, 2008). Trochim and Donnelly (2008) equated reliability in qualitative research with the term dependability. A record was maintained of the evolution of theories, contexts, and generalizations reached throughout the research process. A series of figures regarding various research milestones is included in Appendix D, pp. 407-410.

Trochim and Donnelly (2008) equated external validity with transferability. Learning in the shared understanding context had to be carefully described in detail in order to give potential value for the body of research.

The local respondent population in Northern California could result in conclusions or situations that may not be generalizable. This limitation was resolved through detailed contextual data explanations clarifying situational and organizational norms (Cohen & Crabtree, 2008; Golafshani, 2003). The results are in the last two chapters.

In addressing transferability in medical education, Downing (2003) suggested "evidence of reasonableness of the proposed interpretation" (p. 830). Argyris (2004) advocated a productive mindset that includes transparency and exploring defensive reactions to look beyond the status quo.

The value of a productive mindset in organizational contexts yields a culture of trust, learning, and productivity. The approach was characterized as double loop learning by Harvard professor Chris Argyris as a method for leaders to reason in response to information. In defensive reasoning, staff members seek to avoid errors and suppress negative feelings about them, while productive reasoning leads staff to acknowledge errors and encourage open discussion about errors (Argyris, 1991). Argyris (1991) suggested that learning is beyond problem solving and more than mere motivation. Mohr (2005) highlighted the importance of leadership awareness of the active, double-loop learning style to affect safety results.

As I contemplated Professor Argyris' research, I concluded that aviation flight decks, over time, transformed to an environment where errors were trapped and mitigated instead of hidden or ignored. A productive mindset is safer than one of defensiveness. However, it was really hard for some people, especially those senior in rank or age, to accept juniors pointing out errors. It took time to change.

Through the aforementioned process of clustering, peer-debriefing, reflexivity, and self-journaling (Cohen & Crabtree, 2008; Colaizzi, 1978; Creswell, 2003; Groenewald, 2004; Patton, 2002; Zikmund, 2003), my study led to rich descriptions of the essence of health care professionals' experiences in the context of the described frameworks.

Delimitations

Smedley (2007) noted the time and cost constraints of in-depth interviews. The scope of the proposed study included a time constraint of approximately four months and respondent access due to schedule conflicts. Careful planning and attentive communications mitigated these boundaries.

Geographic limits of the metropolitan Sacramento and San Francisco areas presented another boundary. To condense required travel, scheduling of purposively selected respondents from representative organizations within a close proximity occurred.

Ethical Assurances

Protection from Harm

A non-attributional, blame-free perspective remained during the study (Bagian, 2005; Pawar, 2007). Although there were no known risks in the study, some of the information may have been considered distressing to some people. Unintended disclosure of medical error was a prominent ethical threat that could result in inappropriate harm to an organization, department, or individual.

A stringent process to collect and document data occurred, and the database remains safeguarded to protect private information from unauthorized disclosure. Pseudonyms were used for all respondents in the dissertation manuscript. All quotes were carefully disclosed to participants, and explicit consent and agreement in the context of the manuscript was confirmed. Study guidelines for human subject protection took place in accordance with the human subject protection rules and regulations promulgated by the Department of Health and Human Services. These measures occurred to provide protection from unintended harm.

Informed Consent

No data was collected prior to IRB approval. All 10 respondents signed the written informed consent form (Appendix C, p. 403), including a pledge of confidentiality. As noted above, we treated confidentiality as paramount.

Respondents were provided a clear explanation of the study's goals and potential outcomes. Results of the data analysis and interpretation were shared with respondents as requested to validate and increase credibility. Representatives from participating institutions reviewed and approved the central research question and were given a copy of the interview guide (Appendix A, p. 395) upon request. Upon release of the study, results include the design so readers may determine the study's credibility (Creswell, 2003).

Right to Privacy

The data collected in the study are confidential. Data coding occurred such that individual names are not associated with information. Specific data are only made available to researchers involved with the project. Respondents were given an opportunity to choose not to answer specific interview questions. Respondents had the right to withdraw from the study at any time without penalty.

Honesty with Professional Colleagues

No deception occurred in the study. Presentation of research analysis and discoveries occurred with transparency and honesty. Reflexive field notes include true thoughts and observations, including descriptions of potential bias or preconceptions (Creswell, 2003; Zikmund, 2003). A series of figures illustrating research steps appears in Appendix D, pp. 407-410.

Gawande (2009) asserted:

> "We have a thirty-billion-dollar-a-year National Institutes of Health, which has been a remarkable powerhouse of medical discoveries. But we have no National Institute of Health Systems Innovation alongside it studying how best to incorporate these discoveries into daily practice—no National Transportation Safety Board (NTSB) equivalent swooping in to study failures the way crash

investigators do, no Boeing mapping out the checklists, no agency tracking the month-to-month results." (p. 185)

One reason for writing this book is contemplation of processes and organizations in aviation serving as models of potential learning for health care. I consider it important to address these gaps.

The United States health care community must place delivery at the forefront of its academic and training infrastructure similar to the study of disease and biology in medical schools and pharmacological and therapy research in laboratories. One way is to consider and adopt qualitative methods to collect and interpret data through the theoretical lens of aviation teamwork methods.

The findings and implications in this research study are anticipated to save lives, decrease injuries, and reduce costs. Let's explore further.

Chapter Four

Root Cause Perspective:

More than Mere Problem Solving

One for the Birds

A true story.

Washington, D.C. municipal workers were baffled with frustration. An excessive amount of bird excrement on the Jefferson Memorial looked horrible. The situation led to frequent power washing, which caused undue erosion of the granite structure. Destroying this national treasure was clearly unacceptable. The problem wrought much angst. Senior leaders were upset and demanded authorities implement immediate action. They really didn't know what else to do.

Technicians considered many solutions, including nets, traps, loud noises, and killing the birds. Why wouldn't nets work? Somebody had to protect the birds, and where was the right place to release them? They couldn't be harmed.

It was time. Crews finally decided to come together in cooperation; the teams sought proactive solutions instead of spinning their wheels with reactive fixes.

When the groundskeepers used a *root cause* approach the solution led to a discovery the birds were feeding on spiders, who fed on an unusual number of midge flies hatching through the day because midge larvae grew under the memorial's roofline.

Well, it turns out that the lights were set to illuminate the memorial's roofline, with the timers turning on shortly before twilight. These specific factors created an ideal condition for midge fly mating. After the lights were adjusted, the birds disappeared. No more bird dung; the power washing days were over (Madden, 2005).

Who would have considered midge fly mating as the root cause of granite erosion? This bird problem and its solution illustrate how exploration and analysis of root causes can provide reasonable and lasting solutions. We should apply this lesson in our desires to grow safety in health care as well as in aviation.

In my work as a safety practitioner, the approach has transformed over time to look not at just solving the problem, but to explore underlying details. Instead of just swatting mosquitoes, spraying repellent, or staying under a net, the best way to mitigate a proliferation of pesky mosquitoes is to find and eliminate places where water can collect and stagnate.

Similarly, finding the root causes of errors involves an organizational climate where errors may be reported and their roots examined in such a way that emphasis remains upon the process and environment in which the person operates rather than on a response of blaming another person.

Chernobyl

Reason's (2000) analysis of the Chernobyl tragedy in the Soviet Union highlighted an insufficient open reporting culture in which technicians violated procedure by switching off safety mechanisms and creating conditions that led to a nuclear reactor meltdown. The Chernobyl technicians acted in response to alarms without regard for or understanding of the underlying conditions.

What type of education and training is necessary to prepare the fertile ground of safety culture transformation? Consider how you were educated on teamwork in your organization, and how what you were taught applies to how you approach problems that need to be solved. Was your education of teamwork deliberate and intentional? Or, did you learn on the job, using lessons from respected peers and mentors?

I'm not saying that learning from peers and mentors is bad; my point is that organizational performance could be much better if teamwork methods were introduced early in one's career. Methods stemming from a deliberate, intentional design rather than anecdotal or chance encounters have greater opportunity to produce more thorough and effective teamwork results.

Okay, let's consider another question. Based on teamwork practices from the aviation profession, what value would an open reporting environment yield in health care? Let's explore.

The return on investment to implement teamwork training at an entire hospital is one-tenth the cost of a single wrong-site surgery (Meyers, 2006). A serious malpractice settlement that is avoided pays for CRM-based training tenfold (Ketter, 2006).

The monumental savings in money merits our consideration. We all want to save money, but there are even more visceral reasons to consider these matters.

Catholic Healthcare Partners

At Ohio's largest health provider, Catholic Healthcare Partners, chief executives carry the obituaries of patients in their wallets as a reminder of personal importance. A December 2005 medication error killed a woman undergoing an elective surgery. A retired employee and nurse, the woman also happened to be mother of a high-ranking hospital system executive. As the system's senior leadership observed the anguish and frustration of their colleague, they became impassioned to transform the safety culture at Catholic Healthcare Partners (Crowley & Deen, 2008).

In a commentary five years after the IOM report, health care community leaders noted zero progress had been made and lamented ineffective error reporting systems upon safety (Ferguson & Fakelmann, 2005). Pawar (2007) suggested the most important task for lasting change of service and quality in health care is to facilitate a culture that is free of blame. The conceptual methodology of root cause analysis facilitates exploration of health care's safety culture in an atmosphere free from condemnation.

Root Cause Analysis

Safety advocates use root cause analysis to drill into underlying conditions associated with adverse events (Bagian, 2005; Botwinick et al., 2006; Lu et al., 2006; Reason, 2000; Williams, 2008). Root cause analysis is a subset of systems safety, a methodological approach in safety science founded in the 1960s by scientists in a generation striving to achieve President Kennedy's challenge to walk on the moon.

Systems safety is used by the military to protect nuclear weapons and optimize aerospace projects (Bahr, 1997). Other attributes of systems safety include analysis of hazards and implementation of systematic corrections in response to changing conditions (Bahr, 1997; Lu et al., 2006).

Authors of contemporary management literature and scholarly researchers over the past decade extol the value of culture transformation (Chase & McCarthy, 2010; Ferguson & Fakelmann, 2005; Pronovost et al., 2003). In 2003 U.S. Senate testimony the health care accreditation chair noted an urgent need for reformed medical and nursing education to affect cultural change (The Joint Commission, 2003). For communication improvements, health personnel must resolve cultural barriers related to disclosure of errors, including the relational characteristic of hierarchy (Helmreich, 2000). Sutker (2008) reported health industry communication errors may be attributed to the importance given to individual competency in medical academic training.

Challenger Disaster

In 1986, President Reagan chartered a commission that elucidated safety culture as a key concept in a root cause context in the aftermath of the space shuttle *Challenger* disaster (Bahr, 1997). Poor team communication at NASA influenced pressures to proceed with the launch despite a high-risk condition, leading to a catastrophic fatal explosion (Bahr, 1997; Carroll, Gormley, Bilardo, Burton, & Woodman, 2006). Under pressure from management, safety engineers concurred with the launch in a culture of "fear of ridicule and punishment" (Bahr, 1997, p. 43). Investigators of this tragedy noted four failures (Bahr, 1997):

1. Lack of reporting
2. Poor trend analysis
3. Misrepresented criticality
4. Scarce leader participation in key discussions

Another key systematic flaw at NASA during the *Challenger* disaster was lack of alignment between management layers (Carroll et al., 2006). Most importantly, safety managers were not given authority to render independent system checks and balances (Bahr, 1997).

Aviation safety advocates in the 1960s-era U.S. Air Force noted the importance of organizational culture for error prevention (Martin, 1993; Wood, 2004). The Air Force experienced an unusually high number of engine failures, and investigators noted an interesting problem (Wood, 2004). During a program to obtain oil samples from jet engines to monitor engine wear and extend life, mechanics kept dropping the sample bottles into the oil tanks (Wood, 2004). The diameter of the bottles was an exact fit to plug the supply line to the engines, resulting in an unexpected engine failure and subsequent crash (Wood, 2004).

The Air Force investigated these incidents in organizations in which engine failures continued and found chiefs of these organizations routinely punished the mechanics caught dropping the bottles into the oil tanks (Wood, 2004). Squadron leaders who used a systems approach thanked the technician for reporting the error, a strategy that prevented further engine failures (Wood, 2004). The final solution was simple: the Air Force required bottles larger than the tank opening (Wood, 2004). A more valuable lesson was the positive impact of a systems approach over a blame-oriented approach for permanent culture change rather than temporary action with unintended consequences.

> A more valuable lesson was the positive impact of a systems approach over a blame-oriented approach for permanent culture change rather than temporary action with unintended consequences.

In addition to a systems approach, another process technique to explore root causes is the five whys theory developed by Japanese scholar M. Imai (Pawar, 2007). In the five whys theory, one asserts importance on process over individuals. Pawar (2007) provided an example in which a lack of supplies caused physicians' frustration. Instead of blaming the staff for not doing their job, workers traced the problem to a lack of standard protocols for ordering, receiving, and storing supplies (Pawar, 2007).

The current literature includes evidence that numerous health organizations began implementation of aviation teamwork methods in their patient safety programs because of the aforementioned IOM report (Leape et al., 2009; Musson & Helmreich, 2004; Wachter, 2010). Additional research into the root causes of health industry errors would increase the body of knowledge. Stone et al. (2005) noted a gap in patient safety culture assessment constructs. Pratt et al. (2007) highlighted a lack of scholarly data for clinical outcomes influenced by aviation-based programs.

Empirical data fall short of defining a positive safety culture in health care organizations, but health care researchers agree culture change solutions stem from improved performance and safety initiatives (Fleming & Wentzell, 2008). Fleming and Wentzell (2008) noted the difficulty of using mailed questionnaires to improve safety culture through practical actions. Fleming and Wentzell

(2008) adapted a tool from the petrochemical industry for health care, using a five-phase continuum:

1. Pathological: No systems in place to promote a positive safety culture.
2. Reactive: Systems are piecemeal, developed only in response to occurrences and/or regulatory or accreditation requirements.
3. Calculative: Systematic approach to patient safety exists, but implementation is patchy, and inquiry into events is limited to circumstances surrounding specific events.
4. Proactive: Comprehensive approach to promoting a positive safety culture exists; evidence-based intervention implemented across the organization.
5. Generative: Creation and maintenance of a positive safety culture are central to mission of the organization; organization evaluates the effectiveness of interventions and drains every last drop of learning from failures and successes and takes meaningful action to improve. (p. 12)

> "...health care researchers agree culture change solutions stem from improved performance and safety initiatives (Fleming & Wentzell, 2008)."

Following several years of research and debate within an international steering committee that included a VA physician with NASA astronaut experience, The Joint Commission (2007, p. 2) promulgated nine inaugural patient safety solutions in 2007:

1. Look-alike/sound-alike medication names
2. Patient identification
3. Communication during patient handovers
4. Performance of correct procedure at correct body site
5. Control of concentrated electrolyte solutions
6. Assuring medication accuracy at transitions in care
7. Avoiding catheter and tubing misconnections
8. Single use of injection devices
9. Improved hand hygiene to prevent health care associated infection

We should also note The Joint Commission continues to review and update National Patient Safety Goals.

A Learning Culture

These nine basic elements formed a starting point for development of further solutions; however, missing from the list is the concept of a learning culture. In addition to error resolution, an additional objective of safety culture transformation is to explore root causes of underlying systemic issues associated with errors. A survey on Patient Safety Culture items published by AHRQ (2009) included 12 items:

1. Communication openness
2. Feedback and communication about error
3. Frequency of events reported
4. Handoffs and transitions
5. Management support for patient safety
6. Non-punitive response to error
7. Organizational learning—Continuous improvement
8. Overall perceptions of patient safety

9. Staffing
10. Supervisor/manager expectations and actions promoting safety
11. Teamwork across units
12. Teamwork within units (p. 1-2)

A Learning Culture and Accountability

Accountability is being taken to a new level, a concern for many health organizations, exacerbating the balance between transparency in reporting and disclosure and improvements through culture change (Wachter, 2010). At least 27 U.S. states have reporting requirements for "never events" (Wachter, 2010, p. 3). Researchers from the National Quality Forum launched the list of never events in 2003 and included basic causal factors generally accepted by organizations that theoretically should not occur. This list of eight items has migrated into a "no-pay" (Carpenter, 2007, p. 36) list for Medicare:

1. Falls
2. Heart surgery infections

3. Urinary tract infections resulting from improper use of catheters
4. Pressure ulcers
5. Vascular infections resulting from improper use of catheters
6. Objects left in the body after surgery
7. Air embolisms
8. Blood incompatibility

As a result, the health care industry estimates $20 million in Medicare payment savings (Carpenter, 2007). However, the adverse impacts could result in unnecessary tests and reduced error reporting (Carpenter, 2007). Although 1,285 hospitals agreed to waive billing for a never event, 87% of the same organizations conceded that policies were not in place to prevent the most common health care infections (Carpenter, 2007).

My book isn't intended to take one side or another in the health care debate. I simply want to see errors trapped and mitigated before patients are injured or killed. Under the

Affordable Care Act, Medicare will withhold one percent of payment to hospitals not achieving a baseline score. If the initiative survives the political debate, funds will be redirected to other high-achieving organizations. Given today's budgets and competitive business climate, how might a better understanding of teamwork help your health care organization do a better job? Shall we continue to only swat mosquitoes, power wash granite, and switch off alarms? It's time we worked smarter and achieved more beneficial results.

Please join me as we shift gears and explore how aviation worked to solve underlying hazards on flight decks. These efforts began a long time ago, and I'm convinced their learning value provides opportunity for health care error mitigation. More importantly, I see potential for lasting and sustained safety culture transformation. As you read on, keep your *Befindlichkeit* perspective in mind.

Chapter Five

Aviation Safety's Transformation: Roots of Change

1943 is the year.

If you had to guess, would you think American air forces lost more aircraft and aviators that year in combat, or in non-combat accidents? Were there more losses in Europe, the Pacific, or in the United States?

As battles raged on all fronts, American industry churned out nearly 300,000 airframes during the entire war.

Bombers, transports, fighters, torpedo planes, dive-bombers, training aircraft. Many were flown in non-combat settings by women, who filled vital manpower gaps in the aftermath of standing up a two-front force to face Germany and Japan.

Military senior leadership during World War II understood the importance of conserving precious resources; however, a prevailing philosophy rendered safety secondary to mission (Wood, 2003). Recognition of the relevance and cost benefit of safety led to the creation of aeronautical safety centers at each of the military service branches in the 1950s (Weiner & Nagel, 1998).

Okay, back to our question. Let's answer it.

More than 1,000 more aircraft and aviators were lost in crashes in 1943 in the United States than in combat (Jablonski, 1982; Martin, 1993; Weiner & Nagel, 1988).

There must have been a lot of crashes stateside, because in 1943 the Americans launched massive air raids on

Schweinfurt's ball bearing plants, Ploesti's refineries, and Regensburg's Messerschmitt factories. America suffered great losses at the hand of the Luftwaffe, not to mention Navy and Marine Corps battles in the Pacific.

Why is this fact important? I believe that even mundane, routine, day-to-day losses matter, too. As losses mount, we must count the cost. Not to blame who made the mistake, but to learn from it so we can prevent it next time.

Each one matters. When aggregated in context, we can discern insightful trends. We might even discover a *Befindlichkeit*.

> As losses mount, we must count the cost. Not to blame who made the mistake, but to learn from it so we can prevent it next time.

Mitch Morrison

Roots of Aviation Safety Transformation

Aviation's methods to orchestrate a cohesive safety transformation began over a century ago with America's most lauded aviation pioneers—the Wright Brothers. When Orville Wright and an Army Lieutenant were conducting the final acceptance flight for a prototype military airplane in September 1908, the aircraft suddenly dove into the ground, killing the Lieutenant (Martin, 1993; Stahel, 2008).

Interestingly, the Library of Congress website contains original correspondence between Lieutenant Thomas Selfridge and the Wright Brothers. The Lieutenant sought to promote aviation in the U.S. Army; however, the Wright Brothers were working with the British and French, putting off the Lieutenant. After several months of delays and coordination for the flights, this day had come.

The Army commissioned a board to investigate the cause of the crash and found a newly installed long propeller had contacted a rudder guy wire, leading to the wire coming out of its fitting. The wire failure allowed the rudder assembly to fail, resulting in a catastrophic shift in the aircraft's center of gravity, which caused the dive. The results of this first investigation provided data for the manufacturers (the Wright Brothers) to redesign guy wire locations to remain well clear of propellers.

Today the airlines and military use reporting and analysis in a systems-based environment to mitigate root causes of errors (Reason, 2000; Weiner et al., 1993; Wells & Rodrigues, 2004). Aviation personnel use well-designed checklists and structured briefings and debriefings for crew and passenger safety; however, these process improvements have not been always in place (Pratt et al., 2007).

Investigators of early aviation accidents cited procedure or engineering-related issues as causal factors (Wells & Rodrigues, 2004). The United States Air Mail Service established the first documented safety program designed to prevent mishaps (Wells & Rodrigues, 2004). On a per mile basis, U.S. commercial aviation experienced 34.3 times more mishaps as the Air Mail Service in 1924, and Congress passed the Air Commerce Act of 1926, establishing safety standards for commercial aviation (Wells & Rodrigues, 2004).

As researchers explored the drop in mishap rates because of aviation engineering improvements, attention to human error by industry leaders and accident investigators moved to the forefront. Engineers learned from analysis of material failures to implement robust design characteristics for mechanical redundancy, including the advent of jet-powered aircraft in the late-1950s (Sexton et al., 2000). As these improvements reduced engine and airframe failures, accident investigators discovered human factors to be a new frontier for aviation safety (Sexton et al., 2000).

Birth of the Federal Aviation Administration

In 1956, a midair collision over the Grand Canyon, after sequential departures from Los Angeles of a Chicago-bound United DC-7 and a Kansas City-bound TWA Super

Constellation, killed 128 people (Wells & Rodrigues, 2004). The public called for reform, leading regulators to create the Federal Aviation Administration (FAA) and a system of air traffic management with the Federal Aviation Act of 1958 (Wells & Rodrigues, 2004).

Reforms by legislators led to robust regulatory influence at government and organizational levels, including a cadre of more than 40,000 FAA inspectors by 1961, to conduct pilot check flights and oversee maintenance facilities (Wells & Rodrigues, 2004). Manufacturers began installation of equipment for recording radio and cockpit conversations for investigator analysis (Wells & Rodrigues, 2004).

I think the tipping point to initiate deliberate culture change in aviation's safety culture began as a result of analyzing voice transcripts. The airlines were moving into the jet era, with experienced pilots filling their ranks: new equipment, highly qualified people, a booming economy. Flight deck recording systems provided a new way to respond to crashes.

Eastern 401

In 1972 on approach into Miami, three well-qualified pilots led by a 30,000 flight-hour captain became distracted by a burned out light bulb and allowed a four-month-old Eastern Airlines Lockheed jet to crash during darkness in the Florida Everglades (Weiner et al., 1993). Investigators discovered lack of assertive communications between the pilots and air traffic controllers as a root cause of the crash.

In the voice recorder transcript, the air traffic controller noticed the pilots' descent, asking, "How is everything coming along out there?" A culture of professional deference, not wanting to directly point out mistakes, was present. The pilots had everything under control. They knew what they were doing. They were proud, well-trained, well-equipped.

So, what went wrong?

Distracted by an erroneous landing gear indication brought on by an inexpensive light bulb, the experienced crew all tried at once to fix the problem. Nobody was flying the plane.

At the last second, one of the pilots finally noticed the descent, saying, "Hey! What's going on here?" It was too late to recover the descent.

I want you to note the lack of assertive, clear, accurate, and concise language used by the pilots and air traffic controllers (ATC). A good ATC alert: "Eastern 401, terrain alert, you are descending." And a good pilot response: "We are descending, I have the controls," while adding takeoff power to arrest the descent.

As they began to review accidents, investigators noted alarming trends. These reviews sparked nationwide debate over how aircrews worked together (Musson & Helmreich, 2004).

Tenerife

In March 1977, the deadliest accident in aviation history resulted in 583 deaths on Tenerife in the Canary Islands (Wells & Rodrigues, 2004). Heavily accented air traffic controllers used ambiguous language regarding the position of two aircraft shrouded in fog, and a Dutch Boeing 747 from KLM Airlines on its takeoff roll collided with a taxiing Pan American Airlines Boeing 747 (Weiner et al., 1993).

The voice recorder from the Dutch jet indicated an impatient, hurried captain who failed to confirm the controller's takeoff clearance, despite doubts by other crewmembers (Weiner et al., 1993). Paradoxically, Captain Von Zanten was a high-ranking KLM training pilot whose photo was prominent in corporate advertising (Weiner et al., 1993).

Portland

Describing the 1978 United DC-8 crash in Portland, Oregon, Helmreich (1996) noted authoritarian behavior by the captain and lack of assertiveness by the flight engineer. Insufficient teamwork in handling a simple landing gear malfunction allowed the aircraft to crash due to fuel exhaustion (Helmreich, 1996).

After the United crash in Portland, aviation leaders noted an urgent need to resolve problematic flight deck authority gradients. Did captains listen to co-pilots? Did juniors fear speaking up?

Or... did hierarchy prevail over reason?

Although the problem existed, many suggested that things were fine. They could all just buckle down and do better. Captains defended their position, hiding behind decades of tradition. They had paid their dues. No young first officer or woman flight attendant was telling them how to run their cockpit!

Sound familiar?

> ... did hierarchy prevail over reason?

Finally, leaders collaborated with National Aeronautics and Space Administration (NASA) psychologists to establish an iterative team coordination training process known as Crew Resource Management (CRM) (Weiner et al., 1993). By the mid-1980s, the FAA implemented CRM for scheduled U.S. airline operations, military branches, and many world airlines.

An inherent strength of CRM is crewmembers knowing their roles and responsibilities and interacting through structured communications protocols with little personal familiarity. Other benefits include improved morale and increased operations efficiency. We'll look further into CRM in the next chapter.

As aviation benefited from the cultural changes on flight decks due to safety improvements, a lack of maintenance inspectors became aviation's weak link. In 1996, two maintenance-related crashes within a nine-week period resulted in a White House Commission on Aviation Safety chaired by Vice President Gore (Wells & Rodrigues, 2004).

A Valujet DC-9 crashed into the Florida Everglades when unserviceable oxygen generation gear stored with tires ignited in the cargo hold, resulting in an uncontrollable fire killing 110 aboard (NTSB, 1998b).

TWA Flight 800 exploded shortly after takeoff from New York City, killing 220 when an electrical short circuit in the quantity indicating system caused a fuel tank to explode (NTSB, 2000).

Most of the 1996 commission's discoveries related to aviation security improvements, a chilling harbinger of the vulnerabilities exposed during the September 11, 2001, terrorist attacks (Wells & Rodrigues, 2004).

In January 2000, an Alaska Airlines MD-80 crashed into the ocean north of Los Angeles, caused by an improperly managed maintenance procedure (NTSB, 2003). Lack of lubrication led to a broken elevator jackscrew that rendered the aircraft uncontrollable, killing all 88 aboard (NTSB, 2003). Included in the causal factors in the Valujet, TWA, and Alaska accident reports was lack of airline regulatory oversight by the FAA (NTSB, 2003).

Despite a known lack of inspectors over the past decade, NTSB and FAA actions in 2007 continued to target maintenance management interventions (NTSB, 2007). Reason (2000) noted that 90% of aviation maintenance errors are blameless mistakes and the result of systems management failures.

Aviation has transformed to a systems-oriented process that includes programs designed to work in parallel with one another. I have seen analogies comparing health care losses, one at a time, to aviation losses, where hundreds of lives could be lost in a single tragic mishap. Depending on which losses count in health care, the comparison adds up to an airliner crash with over a hundred on board every other day. This would be unacceptable in aviation.

I believe the numbers and how they are counted remain less important than the mindset. I have seen the aftermath of catastrophic loss in aviation. Everybody wants to do something, to fix the problem. By then, however, for those affected, it's too late.

One thing is certain: whether aviation, health care, or other high stakes pursuit—the next loss matters to *someone*. Therefore, preventing each loss, one at a time, matters to you and me. What can we do now?

Let's strive to understand new ways to prevent and trap errors before consequences occur. The "ounce of prevention is better than a pound of cure" adage comes to mind.

And, that's the point.

We have looked at several examples serving as a spark toward safety culture transformation in aviation. In the next chapter, we'll explore the nuts and bolts of CRM, checklists, briefings, and reporting-analysis, and set the stage for exploring aviation teamwork in health care.

Chapter Six

Aviation Teamwork: Translating Key Tools to Health Care Settings

December 17, 1948

On the forty-fifth anniversary of the Wright brothers' first flight in 1903, President Harry Truman wrote a statement to commemorate the dedication of a new display at the Smithsonian Museum. "Neither the famous brothers nor their contemporaries from forty-five years ago could have realized the importance of this pioneer flight in the subsequent development of aviation and the complete transformation to be wrought in human affairs through mastery of the air."

I like President Truman's comment illustrating the profound impact aviation had already made to transform humanity. The transformation continues.

Orville Wright died earlier in 1948, and his executors worked with the British government to return back the original Wright flyer from London to the United States. In the aforementioned display dedication, astute British Ambassador Sir Oliver Franks quoted from the Wright Brothers' writings: "The best dividends on labor invested have invariably come from seeking more knowledge rather than more power." In concluding the address, Mr. Franks said: "…we must bring to that task what the Wright Brothers brought to theirs, a conviction that what we need above all is knowledge, patience, and courage. I hope that all who see the Kitty Hawk in its permanent home here in the

Smithsonian will be inspired by it to bring to their tasks the qualities which enabled the Wright Brothers to write so notable a first page in the history of man-carrying flight."

These quotes provide a springboard into a discussion of aviation teamwork. Ambassador Franks' comments transcended aviation, politics, and national cultures. I'm struck by an emphasis upon the passion and persistence exuded by Wilbur and Orville Wright. Strong qualities of effort and determination remain in both aviation and health care today. This is common ground as we explore **Teamworks**.

During the past 30 years, aviation's safety culture has transformed to taxonomy of assertive team-oriented communications (McGreevy et al., 2006; Musson & Helmreich, 2004). Aviation teamwork methods are aligned with a systems-based culture in which junior staff members advocate concerns without blame (Bagian, 2005; Conway, 2005) and senior leaders exhibit transparency and openness without fear (Argyris, 2004). Although aviation teamwork methods are not implemented to eliminate errors, the schema result in trapped errors before adverse consequences occur.

Reflect upon this statistic. The influence of aviation's cultural transformation attributed to teamwork improvements from 1987 to 2006 reduced fatal accidents of U.S. scheduled airlines by 74% (NTSB, 2007). As aviation teamwork improved, leaders worked to use other tools for safety. Current initiatives include computerized aircraft monitoring systems and web-based reporting tools. Health care uses similar technology in many settings.

The learning context of this paradigm shift includes aviation teamwork methods represented by four key components: teamwork combined with Crew Resource Management (CRM), checklists, briefings, and open reporting-analysis (Gawande, 2007; Haynes et al., 2009; Weiner et al., 1993). These safety initiatives provide a contextual framework to explore analogous changes in health care in order to mitigate root causes of medical errors. In combination, the four components serve as a contextual framework for my research to compare aviation's transformation with those of health care.

While specific teamwork methods (e.g., reporting or CRM) implemented in aviation are not suggested as a panacea to correct health care's culture immediately, the phenomenon warranted further exploration in medical settings. In 2001 Helmreich, Musson, and Sexton suggested adaptation of aviation's error-tolerant culture in medicine, but highlighted important differences. Sexton et al. (2000) cautioned that implementation of aviation methods "be fully validated to avoid haphazard approaches of limited utility" (p. 749). Musson and Helmreich (2004) noted many solutions available for health care included proprietary content, making them difficult to compare or evaluate regarding clinical benefit.

An increasing number of health organizations are using aviation-based practices to improve teamwork and mitigate medical errors. Fosdick and Uphoff (2007) cited a decrease of average patient days from 6.29 to 5.72 at the Nebraska

Medical Center over a five-year period when aviation-based strategies were used. The results of aviation teamwork implementations revealed clinical improvements; however, the best programs required careful tailoring, significant leadership commitment, and took time (12-18 months) for manifestation of measurable results.

As in any technical task, follow up refresher training is essential to sustain beneficial change. As desired behavior is modeled, practiced, and taught, the desired outcomes will result. Sadly, many organizations may not be willing to invest the required resources for culture transformation (Crowley & Deen, 2008).

Helmreich (2000) noted a lack of key behaviors to mitigate risk and errors in operating rooms, including communication, leadership, conflict resolution, and vigilance. Without communication, team integrity fails. Without leadership, individuals struggle. Without conflict resolution, divisions remain and teachable moments are lost. Without vigilance, people lose focus.

I believe that scholars are correct to assert that significant research is necessary to understand effective implementation of aviation teamwork methods in health care to inspire safety culture transformation (Looseley, Houtouras, & Keogh, 2009; Lyndon, 2008; Thomas, 2006). Exploration of root causes for medical error extends to foundations and methods of patient safety education for health care staffs. As research efforts continue, we have opportunity to save lives, decrease injuries, and reduce costs. These are worthy goals, and we should pursue them.

When viewed in a community-wide context, aviation's safety culture transformation is more developed as compared to health care's safety culture transformation (Leape et al., 2009; Musson & Helmreich, 2004). That said, I think health care is making strides. In the end, both communities offer tremendous opportunity to transform in a shared spiral of learning and understanding. Visualize a pinnacle, where each community endeavors a climb to the top. Each group shares information on best practices, helping the other map the best route. Together, they achieve much more collectively than they could individually.

You may have noticed that I refer to aviation teamwork in different contexts. I use three different terms:
1. Aviation Teamwork Methods
2. Aviation Teamwork Heuristics
3. Aviation Teamwork Ontology

I think aviation methods stem from heuristics, or rules of thumb. Scholars sometimes use the term *cognition* to describe a process of knowledge creation. Used over time, these processes create an ontology, or permanent transformational change. In simpler terms:
1. Methods: what we do
2. Heuristics: what we know
3. Ontology: who we are

As we continue, let's reflect again upon our *Befindlichkeit*. What skills and behaviors do you practice, based upon what you know, to transform your core being toward teamwork and safety?

Aviation Teamwork Heuristic

The Aviation Teamwork Heuristic (ATH) is an interpretive, mutually interdependent framework characterizing the eureka-like discovery of a dynamic process of shared responsibility, community (e.g., aviation or health care) transformation, learning, and adaptation. The foundation for the ATH is the evolution of these team-oriented concepts in aviation: CRM, checklists, briefings, and reporting-analysis. Double loop learning remains another concept associated with these methods.

Double Loop Learning

The phenomenological foundation of aviation's culture transformation includes double loop learning (Argyris, 2002; Mohr, 2005; Senge et al., 1994). Argyris (1991) conceptualized double loop learning as an organizational strategy to transform attitudes and behaviors beyond problem solving.

Picture the first loop as fixing or resolving a problem. The second loop is going back to explore underlying aspects of what caused the problem. Argyris described the single loop as mere problem solving and described ignoring the source of the problem as a doom loop.

Argyris (1991) further described the doom loop as defensive reasoning and suggested that people often confuse learning as problem-solving in both organizational and individual contexts. Looking back to the Chernobyl example, this illustrates the single loop; the Shuttle *Challenger* example illustrates the doom loop (Argyris, 1991). In Chernobyl, the technicians switched off the alarms, ignoring their source (single loop). In *Challenger*, leadership ignored the source of the problem (doom loop).

Argyris (1991) suggested productive reasoning is necessary to achieve double loop transformation. When organizations implement a paradigm of productive reasoning or double loop learning, errors, near misses, and hazards are opportunities for improvement rather than events for people to fear (Leape et al., 2009; Mohr, 2005). Argyris' (1991) double loop learning concept is analogous with aviation's pilot and flight deck culture transformation, achieved through CRM, checklists, briefings, and open reporting-analysis. The double loop pedagogy is a conceptual foundation for the theoretical framework of aviation teamwork methods and potential applicability in health care.

Crew Resource Management (CRM)

In a survey of 125 medical centers at the Veteran's Administration, researchers noted a "strong correlation between teamwork culture across professional disciplines and patient satisfaction" (Dunn et al., 2007, p. 318). Clancy and Tornberg (2007) noted difficulty of the health care community adopting a teamwork science because health care professionals are "trained to function as individuals in hierarchical arrangements" (p. 215). Musson and Helmreich (2004) concluded CRM training was a new concept for health care and suggested development by medical professionals to resolve gaps in coherent implementation guidelines. Salas et al. (2009) noted a small number of curricula include training in teamwork methods. Pratt et al. (2007) also noted little research is available giving evidence on how CRM affects clinical outcomes.

When viewed in a context of historicity, publication of *To Err is Human* in 1999 is analogous to the 1979 NASA Crew Resource Management (CRM) workshop that initiated pilot culture change. The 1999 Institute of Medicine (IOM) report demonstrated the ubiquity of medical error to the health care community (Kohn et al., 1999).

A similar epiphany in aviation occurred in 1982, as the National Transportation Safety Board (NTSB) was forming its Human Performance Division. Air Florida Flight 90 crashed shortly after takeoff in a snowstorm from Washington's National Airport (Weiner et al., 1993). The cockpit voice recorder highlighted poor communications between the pilots (Weiner et al., 1993):

> 1559:58, FIRST OFFICER: God, look at that thing. That doesn't seem right, does it?
>
> 1600:05, FIRST OFFICER: Ah, that's not right...
>
> 1600:09, CAPTAIN: Yes it is, there's eighty. (Captain referring to 80 knots ground speed)
>
> 1600:10, FIRST OFFICER: Naw, I don't think that's right.
>
> 1600:19, FIRST OFFICER: Ah, maybe it is.
>
> 1600:21, CAPTAIN: Hundred and twenty.
>
> 1600:23, FIRST OFFICER: I don't know. (p. 297)

The crew had been sitting on the ground for more than two hours due to winter weather, leading to the formation of ice on the wings and engine probes (Weiner et al., 1993). Failure of the flight crew to activate the engine anti-ice system led to an engine torque probe freezing over and giving the erroneous indication questioned by the first officer during the takeoff roll (Weiner et al., 1993). NTSB causal factors cited failure of the crew to use the engine anti-ice, the captain's indecision, and the first officer's lack of assertiveness to reject the takeoff when faulty indications were noted (Weiner et al., 1993).

NTSB investigators presented data on this accident, and board member J. Lauber noted that making CRM training a requirement would not have prevented the crash (Weiner et al., 1993). However, aviation finally had "come to grips with interaction problems between the captain and first officer" (Weiner et al., 1993, p. 298). Attitudes and behaviors resulting from CRM training, including an assertive first officer and a captain responsive to input, were among the missing factors that led to culture transformation (Weiner et al., 1993).

Assertiveness in an atmosphere of respect and acceptance, where input is welcomed for the safety of any mission, is a natural outcome of aviation-style teamwork. In an environment of trust, personnel exude team behavior as a by-product of their transformative change continuum brought forth from a strong leadership culture.

This is the **Teamworks** philosophy.

A milestone success of CRM occurred in 1989, when a United DC-10 flying from Chicago to Denver experienced metallurgic failure of a turbine wheel in the center engine, causing an explosion that severed all hydraulic lines to the flight control system (Weiner et al., 1993). The flight's Captain used CRM to work together with two other pilots to coax the crippled jet to a miraculous crash landing in Sioux City, Iowa, on a cornfield adjacent to the airport (Wells & Rodrigues, 2004). Team-oriented actions by the crew of United flight 232 saved 184 of 296 passengers aboard (Wells & Rodrigues, 2004). Given this scenario in training simulations, none of the pilots could land safely (A. C. Haynes, personal communication, January 4, 2004). Adding to the success in Sioux City was a recent airport training exercise and National Guard troops on drill status at the airport at the time of the mishap (A. C. Haynes, personal communication, January 4, 2004).

The cognitive errors targeted by CRM include slips, lapses, fumbles, mistakes, and procedure violations (Reason, 2000). Helmreich described the five-phase evolution of aviation CRM in a 1996 symposium. The focus of initial aviation CRM programs included situational awareness, communications, assertiveness, and risk management (Weiner et al., 1993). Follow-on phases included error management, threat mitigation, adaptability and flexibility, and organizational culture (Helmreich, 1996).

In a continuum of understanding, these synthesized programs contribute toward the current revolution of culture transformation. I think aviation must continue its efforts to improve teamwork by transforming processes in maintenance, scheduling, and assigning missions. The next steps include integrated predictive models to assess risk on a daily basis.

When aviation teamwork methods are applied in health care, practitioners must apply operational relevance to the setting, including awareness of organizational and regional culture (Baker et al., 2006). Healey, Undre, and Vincent (2006) asserted teamwork skills were of limited benefit unless linked to tasks and context. Some pilots early in CRM's implementation discounted the relevance of teamwork and rejected the practices as psychobabble (Weiner et al., 1993). Similar resistance is evident in health care implementations. But reflect for a moment on the logic of linking teamwork skills to tasks and content. The **Teamworks** model fits because teams are composed of people acquainted with tasks and the context in which their tasks are performed. It is illogical to reject this truth.

An important element of CRM is teaching crewmembers how to assert safety concerns and challenge and respond to errors (Musson & Helmreich, 2004). Researchers noted concerns with CRM training in health care without adaptation (Musson & Helmreich, 2004; Salas et al., 2006). Salas et al. (2006) asserted that company-specific CRM programs do not export seamlessly to other organizations or industries. Dunn et al. (2007) noted the key role non-clinician faculty members have in "translating CRM relevance from aviation to health care" (p. 321). Recurrent CRM concepts are vital for organizational success, but sometimes were forgotten or ignored over time by some uninterested participants (Helmreich, 1996).

I want to define the authority gradient. Picture in your mind a line in graph form from the senior person (Captain) to the junior person (First Officer or Co-Pilot). In aviation's old days the slope was steep; however, now, it is much shallower. Someone must remain in command, but the pedestal isn't too high. Co-pilots can speak and be heard. Captains encourage crew assertiveness and innovation rather than deference and compliance.

Consider one example of leaders who mitigated the authority gradient of airline captains working with first officers, flight attendants, mechanics, and dispatchers in aviation's culture transformation (Musson & Helmreich, 2004). In January 1989, investigators' reports of a Boeing 737 crash in Britain illustrated a lack of teamwork both inside and outside the flight deck (Besnard, Greathead, & Baxter,

2003; Hamman, 2004). While flying from London to Belfast, the crew experienced heavy vibration and smoke in the cockpit and the co-pilot incorrectly identified the perceived source (Besnard et al., 2003). In haste to eliminate the vibration and smoke, the captain reduced power to initiate a descent and directed the co-pilot to shut down the right engine on the twin-engine jet (Besnard et al., 2003). The combined actions of reduced power on the left engine and shutdown of the right engine resulted in decreased vibration and elimination of smoke (Besnard et al., 2003). The cabin flight crew and some passengers were aware of sparks and flames emanating from the left engine, but this information was not communicated to the pilots (Besnard et al., 2003). As the pilot increased power on the left engine to arrest the descent for landing, the left engine failed, causing a stall that plunged the stricken jet into a hill just short of the East Midlands airport, killing 39 and injuring 74 others (Besnard et al., 2003).

The British Midlands case illustrates the relevance of open communication between all crew members, accepting cues from passengers, and processing the data for a coherent decision. Analogically, medical staff must communicate through varied levels and accept patient input as applicable. In health care, the authority gradient of all staff, including physicians teaming with residents, nurses, anesthesiologists, other specialists, and patients is even more complex than in aviation.

For example, Aggarwal, Undre, Moorthy, Vincent, and Darzi (2004) stated surgery is 25% dexterity and 75% decision-making. Kosnik, Brown, and Maund (2007) described how CRM-based teamwork among nurses changed communications, decision making, and implementation of technology. Like aviation, the team worked together with assertiveness and innovation rather than deference and compliance. Staff at the Nebraska Medical Center conducted CRM-based training over a three-day period with strong participation from physicians and nurses (Meyers, 2006). Meyers also found that at the end of the training, the board supported widespread implementation.

Adapted CRM in health care is a convergence of team coordination and error trapping, shaped by systems safety strategies and influenced by best practices from the quality philosophies. The cost for a private vendor to implement CRM at a large hospital was $100,000 to $200,000, and $60,000 to $80,000 at a smaller hospital (Meyers, 2006). Teamwork training for 1,045 staff at the Nebraska Medical Center (NMC) resulted in a J.D. Power award for two consecutive years (Fosdick & Uphoff, 2007). Six-Sigma and supply chain management were two non-aviation methods used at NMC (Fosdick & Uphoff, 2007).

Marshall and Manus (2006) reported the impact of human factors training at five hospitals using CRM-based concepts, noting 12 dimensions:
1. Overall Perceptions of Safety
2. Frequency of Events Reported
3. Supervisor/Manager Expectations and Actions Promoting Patient Safety
4. Organizational Learning/Continuous Improvement.
5. Teamwork within Units

6. Communication Openness
7. Feedback and Communication about Error
8. Non-punitive Response to Error
9. Staffing
10. Hospital Management Support for Patient Safety
11. Teamwork across Hospital Units
12. Hospital Handoffs and Transitions (p. 996-997)

A 12-step survey was used before and after implementation of training protocols, with an increase of 7.4% in the 12 dimensions from the Hospital Survey on Patient Safety Culture, a standardized survey developed by researchers from the Agency of Health Care Research and Quality (Marshall & Manus, 2006).

A lack of engagement by physicians was a key factor, mitigated by use of peers and internal physician champions (Marshall and Manus, 2006). Marshall and Manus (2006) noted deeply embedded traditions of autonomy and fear of lost authority, which represented impediments to culture change. Similarly, Ferguson and Fakelmann (2005) noted the following barriers: "Premium placed on autonomy and perfection; cooperation and communications are lacking; mistakes are treated as personal and professional failure; teamwork and collaboration in problem solving are poor" (p. 40).

In 2001, Harvard University's Beth Israel Deaconess Medical Center (BIDMC) was one of the first in health care and the first in obstetrics to apply CRM in clinical medicine practice (Pratt et al., 2007). A randomized study explored team training's effects on health-related outcomes in 14,271 deliveries from 1999-2001 and 19,380 deliveries from 2003-2006 (Pratt et al., 2007). Pratt et al.'s (2007) analysis of malpractice data from the two periods revealed a drop in cases from 21 to 16 lawsuits, with a 62% drop from 13 to five in the high severity category. After implementation of teamwork protocols, Pratt et al. (2007) concluded that almost 300 less women experienced adverse outcomes.

During implementation of aviation teamwork methods, BIDMC invested time and effort to tailor the program specifically to their organization and created an in-depth four-tier module explaining teamwork skills (Pratt et al., 2007). All personnel attended mandatory team training, dedicated staff members conducted e-mail campaigns and meetings, and leaders praised team members who publicly used the new techniques (Pratt et al., 2007). Initial measures over a short time failed to reveal a change of outcomes; however, when managers placed a persistent emphasis during a period of 12 months, a significant positive effect was noted (Pratt et al., 2007). As management presented the positive outcomes to the staff, the positive trends increased commitment and reinforced a new culture at BIDMC (Pratt et al., 2007).

It is exciting to see a cutting edge implementation at a high-profile health care provider. These changes sparked the roots of culture transformation, which could be emulated in many other places. From a practical standpoint, almost a patient a day escaped the consequences of error; directly attributed to aviation teamwork methods!

In 2006 the Vanderbilt University Medical Center (VUMC) in Nashville achieved a safety rating in the top 10 of 900 U.S. hospitals after training leaders in team communications, decision-making, performance feedback, fatigue countermeasures, and wrong-site surgery (Ketter). Vanderbilt's program trained more than 2,700 staff and implemented CRM methods in four hospitals (Ketter, 2006). A gap noted in the Vanderbilt program is adherence to 24-hour shifts by physicians, despite recognition of the adverse impacts of fatigue (Ketter, 2006). One return on investment for Vanderbilt's program was eradication of wrong-site surgery, despite 35,000 to 40,000 annual procedures (Ketter, 2006). Vanderbilt's implementation staff included two former astronaut physicians and a former U.S. Air Force physiologist (The Joint Commission, 2006).

The University of Utah used prior military instructors to teach medical residents in a systems approach, abandoning an autonomous "supreme, captain-of-the-ship" environment (McGreevy et al., 2006, p. 1083). Clancy and Tornberg (2007) introduced a Department of Defense-sponsored program entitled "TeamSTEPPS—Team Strategies and Tools to Enhance Performance and Patient Safety" (p. 214). Alonso et al. (2006) described implementation of TeamSTEPPS in numerous military hospitals to mitigate errors. Lyndon (2008) explained challenges with the "traditional hierarchical structure of medicine" (p. 18) and a tendency of nurses to avoid conflict.

Current literature cites difficulty in implementing community-wide CRM-based concepts. Qualitative methods are appropriate to define how team initiatives mitigate medical errors. I agree with any research method, quantitative or qualitative, to measure the long-term effectiveness of teamwork upon clinical outcomes. Shall we wait to see the evidence or begin immediately to roll up our sleeves and work together on solutions?

Let's continue to look at another defined structure provided to personnel to optimize management of complex procedures.

Checklists

A Joint Commission study of errors from 1995 to 2003 concluded that 76% were wrong site, 13% wrong person, and 11% wrong procedure (Chodroff, 2007). Checklists provide a leading solution for wrong site events (Chodroff, 2007). They are used in many medical applications, including prevention of medication errors, which harm 1.5 million people and cause approximately 7,000 U.S. deaths (Kliger et al., 2009). Clearly, checklists are important.

The origin of checklists in aviation precedes World War II. In October 1935, during a competition in Ohio for the next generation bomber, an experienced Army test pilot executed a takeoff in an aluminum prototype Boeing 299 with the control lock engaged, resulting in a crash that killed two of five crewmembers (Gawande, 2007). Dubbed the "Flying Fortress" by a Seattle journalist, the complex bomber had four engines, retractable landing gear, hydraulically controlled propellers, and other modern systems for the pilot to manage (Gawande, 2007). Government and civilian executives feared the aircraft was more than man could handle, but a group of test pilots collaborated on a simple reference booklet to standardize procedures and called it a checklist (Gawande, 2007). Despite a dismal safety record over the following years, the Air Corps pilots used their checklists and never experienced another control lock crash in over 1.8 million flight miles with 13,000 B-17 airframes to defeat Nazi Germany (Gawande, 2007).

In 2001, a physician created a checklist for insertion of central lines into the chest of patients, a "lifeline for delivering medication that becomes infected in four percent of cases" (Barlow, 2008, p. 28). In 2003, the same physician researched correlations of infection by following five core checklist steps in 100 Michigan hospitals (Barlow, 2008). In the initial phase of the study, researchers noted that 30% of staff skipped one of the steps; however, after 15 months of using the checklist, the rate of infection dropped to zero, saving 1,500 lives and almost $200 million (Barlow, 2008). Release of the 2006 study by the World Health Organization included a sample 19-step checklist (Barlow, 2008).

My first experience with aviation checklists was TH-55A helicopter pilot training in the Army. On my first day flying the "Mattel Messerschmidt," I was a nervous 19-year-old who needed a guide to complete simple preflight tasks and before starting engines procedures. Following tradition, at the end of the flight I gave a Jefferson nickel from my birth year to the instructor, signifying my "nickel ride."

In every airframe I've flown, from helicopters to airplanes, a checklist aided safe operation. In most cases, the best practice either mandates or strongly encourages checklists. Checklists work for many processes, not just aviation.

Following this model, use of checklists in health care is growing. In 2011, I had reconstructive thumb surgery. A nurse assistant brought in a checklist, showed it to me, and asked me what I was there for. I told her. Continuing to review the listed items, the surgeon came in and put his signature on the surgical site. When complete, he asked me to confirm he had signed the correct spot. It was very encouraging to see for myself medicine following this practice, just like I did when flying a helicopter or airplane.

It's just as important or even more so when a provider provides complex care for my child. I like the idea of a checklist or job guide to assist, instead of relying solely on memory.

Do we really want to leave things to chance? What do you think?

Based on my examples, we have demonstrated that aviation checklists are well vetted and easy to understand. However, health care has varied facilities, processes, and staff, with more potential for confusion. In a 2009 study, prescribing errors (39%) and medication administration errors (38%) were almost equally distributed (Kliger et al. 2009). When managers implemented checklists to mitigate errors in seven San Francisco hospitals, accuracy improved from 85% to 92% in six months, and to 98% in 18 months (Kliger et al., 2009). A key success factor noted in this project was investment into clinician skills (Kliger et al., 2009). Lancelot (2007) projected cost savings of $2,000 for each adverse drug event, and estimated an automated system to prevent drug errors that, if fully implemented, would avoid up to $2 billion in waste. Checklists are used in conjunction with briefing protocols, the next step in the aviation teamwork methods continuum (Gawande, 2007; Musson & Helmreich, 2004).

Briefings

The most frequent root cause of surgical errors is ineffective communication (Stahel, 2008). To improve communication, aviation organizations have institutionalized briefings, the practice of "short synopses of intended actions" (Musson & Helmreich, 2004, p. 26) prior to flight, during critical operations, and post-flight to critique crew actions. McGreevy et al. (2006) described briefings as a shared mental model of a procedure. Powell and Hill (2006) asserted that a loss of non-verbal cues attributed to surgical masks complicates the health care environment.

Let's define communication. According to author Glen Aubrey in *Core Teams Work: Their Principles and Practices* (p. 127), "Communication is sharing information that promotes behavioral change, the results of which become known to appropriate parties. Communication is not fully completed unless behaviors change, hopefully for the better."

Potential briefing items in the health setting include the "SBAR—(Situation, Background, Assessment, Recommendation/Request)" (Kosnik et al, 2007, p. 29), and the time-out, where participants pause for confirmation of critical steps during procedures to confirm elements of nine steps approved by The Joint Commission. Stahel (2008) noted that 85% of surgeon communication errors involved verbal communications, whereas only 4% were written communications, suggesting a read-back procedure to mitigate errors, similar to that in aviation.

Leaders at the BIDMC in Boston used their own staff (instead of outside consultants) to implement briefing protocols to improve team communications and reduced high severity adverse events by 62% (Pratt et al., 2007). Mann, Marcus, and Sachs (2006) presented a briefing process of handing off information from one shift to another, using the acronym SWAP: "Summary of patients; Workload resource management; Abnormal physical findings and lab values; Plan of care" (p. 40). Kosnik et al. (2007) noted blame-free debriefings as an important learning aspect of health organizations. Walton (2006) asserted a need for shifting from "who did it to what happened" (p. 230). Fosdick and Uphoff (2007) highlighted good catches because of time out briefings at the Nebraska Medical Center.

Aviation uses a conflict resolution strategy known as the two challenge rule—a pre-briefed communication protocol where an error is first verbalized by a team member and upon the second challenge without a response the team member will intervene to mitigate the condition (Mann et al., 2006). In health care, nurses and physicians learn different communication techniques; nurses generally provide broad, narrative descriptions to avoid making diagnoses, while physicians tend to be concise (Leonard, Graham, et al., 2004).

Kaiser Permanente hospital in Orange County, California, implemented embedded tools and behaviors for briefings that yielded effective clinical results (Leonard, Graham, et al., 2004). I think briefings are important for staff moving toward or away from tasks or situations.

Horwitz, Krumholz, Green, and Huot (2006) cautioned 60% of programs teaching resident physicians were not conducting training in sign-out skills to affect transfers between wards or shifts. Despite the outcome improvements from formalized sign-out programs, a survey of 324 accredited programs revealed continuity gaps due to a lack of technology or lack of explicit means of staff notification (Horwitz et al., 2006). Systems improvements in briefing protocols may adopt "transparency, standardization, and team training" (Hamman, 2004, p. i72). In a Johns Hopkins initiative, researchers implemented Intensive Care Unit (ICU) team briefings that involved shared planning and common goals, resulting in 95% of staff understanding objectives and reducing patient stay lengths from 2.2 days to 1.1 days (Powell, 2007).

This is what the literature says about communication, and my field research confirmed the need for various communities learning communications skills and tools. I'll give several examples in the segments to come.

The fourth phase in the aviation teamwork methods continuum is reporting and analyzing errors in a non-attribution environment. A non-attribution environment is an environment without blame for errors, where one can disclose information without fear of retribution.

Reporting-Analysis

In a study comparing incident reporting in aviation with health care, Powell and Hill (2006) noted that 95% of aviation staff reported errors, but estimated that only 5% of health care staff reported errors (Powell & Hill, 2006). A 2008 survey by the AHRQ reviewed patient safety program input from 108,621 hospital staff members in 2007, and 160,176 hospital staff members in 2008 (AHRQ, 2009).

Areas most in need of improvement included overall reporting and non-punitive response to error (AHRQ, 2009).

Consider how important a non-punitive reporting and response environment is. If every time someone made a mistake they were punished or reprimanded, how would an organization expect opportunity to transform? If you were the one doing the reporting, what would a non-punitive environment provide for you?

Think about this answer: you would settle in and do your job, not looking over your shoulder. You would not perform your duties in complacency or apathy, but with professionalism and collaboration to resolve systems issues, and you would not strive to nit-pick individual differences. This balance is difficult to achieve, because it requires trust built over time. There are no short cuts here.

Aviation began work on this problem decades ago. In 1974, poor communications between air traffic control and pilots of a TWA jet led to a crash near Washington, DC

(Orlady, 1993). Investigators discovered that six weeks prior, a United Airlines crew had reported a similar problem in a newly implemented United Airlines internal reporting system; however, there was no industry-wide process to disseminate the information (Guise, Lowe, & Connell, 2008). As a result, the FAA created the Aviation Safety Reporting System (ASRS), a confidential, non-punitive nationwide system to report hazards (Guise et al., 2008; Wells & Rodrigues, 2004). NASA staff operate the ASRS program and the FAA provides funding (Guise et al., 2008). The ASRS program's goals are to circulate lessons for prevention and to stimulate research; however, confidentiality and system complexity complicate direct response efforts (Orlady, 1993). Although direct response efforts are difficult, researchers may review the data to detect strong trends across specific aircraft models, geographic areas, or technical communities (Orlady, 1993).

Supported by a grant in 2001 from the National Institutes for Health (NIH), a former FAA attorney wrote a white paper for Columbia University outlining the concept of a just culture (Marx, 2001). Marx (2001) noted positive steps in aviation prevention, in which employees reported mistakes in a system free of blame or attribution. In health care, the gamut of behavior includes willful or reckless misconduct, negligent conduct, known violations, and unintentional actions (Marx, 2001; Reason, 2000). Bagian (2005) captured situations in which errors of associated causal factors diverge from an appropriate standard of medical care, including criminal acts, use of alcohol or drugs, or purposefully unsafe actions. Crime, alcohol or drugs, or intentional harm are the limiting situations, which warrant punishment in a safety program (Bagian, 2005). Unfortunately, in response to even unintentional actions, physicians use "denial, discounting, and distancing" (Aron & Headrick, 2002, p. 171), reflective of an accountability culture incompatible with error tolerance.

When denial, discounting, and distancing techniques are used in any team or workgroup atmosphere we can expect errors to be hidden and feared. When lives are at stake, this is dangerous. Regardless, it is not acceptable in any productive environment. To pursue culture transformation, we all must become better.

Military safety programs established strict protections for information gathered during investigations to be used in a privileged manner for learning without retribution (U.S. Air Force, 2004). These open and transparent investigating philosophies yielded a high degree of safety awareness in U.S. commercial and military aviation (Baker et al., 2006; Hamman, 2004; NTSB, 2009). Beyea (2007) highlighted the problem of significant underreporting of wrong-site, wrong patient, and wrong procedure surgery events. Garbutt et al. (2007) researched data from 1,082 doctors and concluded that inadequate reporting systems precluded dissemination of lessons learned. Less than 20% of physicians believed systems to pass on lessons were adequate, and only 30% thought the systems to receive reports were adequate (Garbutt et al., 2007). A root cause of the reporting challenge in health care is that senior doctors were not trained in an era of open reporting (Leape et al., 2009).

Under the leadership of a physician with unique experience as a NASA astronaut, the VA implemented reporting processes for risk assessment and mitigation (Bagian, 2005; DeRosier, Stalhandske, Bagian, & Nudell, 2002). A key element of the VA program is a system that advocates a blameworthy response to protect against unwarranted punishment (Bagian, 2005).

"Blameworthy" means that people are only blamed when appropriate, in isolated instances. Helmreich, Klinect and Wilhelm (1999) outlined five error types (p. 679):

1. Intentional noncompliance errors
2. Procedural errors (slips, lapses, mistakes)
3. Communication errors
4. Proficiency errors
5. Operational decision errors

Sometimes leaders and staff misunderstand culpability for errors, which inhibits safety. In the aforementioned list, after healthy understanding of mitigating pressures and influences, only intentional noncompliance errors merit blame.

The human factors engineering approach to root cause analysis seeks to move beyond asking, "Whose fault is it?" (Bagian, 2005, p. 4) to instead answering, "What happened and why?" and "What can we do to fix it?" (Bagian, 2005, p. 4). However, moving beyond problem analysis to solutions was important to the VA, and reported incidents and near misses increased 30-fold due to an open, blame-free reporting environment (Bagian, 2005).

Critical data were used in a systems perspective to mitigate hazards and reduced errors (Bagian, 2005). Chase and McCarthy (2010) reported VA initiatives emphasized rich understanding of communication through checklists and briefings and debriefings, and they cited an internal report that 80% of VA hospitals had improved patient safety programs (Chase & McCarthy, 2010). Although VA leaders originally thought external reporting had utility, a reduction to only 500 external reports, combined with the unexpected successful collection of 700,000 reports via internal reporting systems, led to cancellation of a contract with NASA to administer the external VA program (Chase & McCarthy,

2010). Culture transformation efforts initiated several years prior were finally taking hold (Chase & McCarthy, 2010).

Given the historical basis and discovery context of the aviation teamwork methods model in comparison with health care initiatives from the current literature, we have a clearly defined point of entry into the hermeneutic circle. This framework provides a basis for interpretative research to improve understanding of root causes of medical errors. Plus, in overall results, we can be gratified that we confirm not only corrective actions for errors, but the underlying systemic aspects that spur transformation in organizations.

Our inquiry will transition into learning what health care people had to say about their experiences with aviation teamwork methods. Before we do so, the next chapter will present more background into my own *Befindlichkeit* to create the ontology argument and framework.

My learned experiences convinced me that what I had experienced for almost 30 years in aviation represented in itself a framework, a perspective to objectively assess health care's transformation. In my literature review, I read about frustration and division in health care, yet admired the intellect, commitment, and passion among physicians, nurses, and other providers.

I wanted to understand health care's transformation on a personal level, yet as a practitioner, all I could offer was my aviation-based teamwork expertise. I wondered, even feared: would these two divergent perspectives yield discovery?

Chapter Seven

Bridging Aviation Teamwork:

From Theories to Field Research

The science of ontology (your *Befindlichkeit*) lends opportunity for error mitigation in aviation, health care, and other high stakes pursuits. If we want to reduce losses in high stakes or high risk endeavor, then we need to get right to the core of one's existence.

When I began my research, I knew this to be true, but lacked evidence to support my assertion. In this short segment, I will explain my journey to create a theoretical model to close the elusive gap between intuition and evidence.

Quality efforts, too often, have become a series of graphs and measures to capture favorable trends rather than an acknowledgement of gutsy and courageous efforts of hardworking professionals. Excellence is measured by the absence of error rather that the toil of a physician, nurse, or other health care professional to introspectively learn the necessary lessons of humility.

Everyone knows they make errors, but the roots of errors aren't measured easily. Investigating them is no small undertaking, but it is a necessary one when the risks and rewards are high.

Concluding that we agree that error mitigation is worth the effort, we must also conclude that understanding safety culture transformation begins with exploring the roots of error mitigation. At the core of this endeavor, two human virtues come into play: it takes *humility* to explore what we don't know that may upon discovery force us, if we're honest, to consider changing our conduct.

Moments of Discovery

The following text includes edited excerpts from my research journal. These excerpts illustrate milestones of my own learning. These moments of discovery helped to frame the theories embedded throughout the book that I applied in the field to collect data.

In phenomenology and hermeneutics, it's my role to use critical theory to detect ideology and culture; to find the implicit versus the explicit. By clarifying matters, my role in this book is to help you make choices.

And, it's still your choice, as it is my choice as well. I discover and give the information from my own perspective that allows you, me, and other interested parties to come to personal conclusions. Choices follow conclusions. They always do.

> Choices follow conclusions. They always do.

When taking field notes, I was careful not to lose the connection between the lived experiences and the mechanical representation of the written words. This goal and mindset forms the basis of entry into the hermeneutical spiral—our collective understanding.

My identity as a researcher is constructivist in a theoretical context. This means that I thrive on exploring the construction process of generating knowledge. I want to understand the why and how behind what people and organizations do to change what they know to transform what they become.

Through a robust body of literature collected during coursework, I formed a perspective that safety and teamwork fundamentals need to be built into educational foundations. I suspected that current teaching methods in health care involve passive consumption through a traditional approach regarding teamwork. The practice was anecdotal or life-skills based instead of an empirical or deliberate approach.

As I ventured into both qualitative science (with understanding), qualitative inquiry with critical theory (ideology), and postmodern thought (constructivist: built knowledge of teamwork), I formed a goal of giving a provisional interpretation as a basis for further research. You may see this goal manifested throughout my work: the root word "interpret" is included in the interpretive phenomenology design.

Let me state this differently: a goal of provisional interpretation is achieved when I can collect data in such as way that it brings forth not only learning or knowledge, but it achieves individual and collective transformation. Related to *Befindlichkeit*, we find ourselves as a community of researchers discovering "Aha" moments that we can share in a spiral of understanding.

My "Aha" moment came when I arrived at this conclusion: I could interpret the findings through a hermeneutic circle context of aviation's transformation. I literally drew and highlighted a light bulb in my journal to illustrate this moment of discovery. Here's the entry:

> "Shank noted the hermeneutic perspective is focused on individual in role as interpreter struggling to make sense of world as found, meaning is based on continuum of where culture is interpreted (in eyes of researcher). Patton asserted the cultural context includes where the data were created and where (also) it is interpreted. The historical context of applied aviation methods places the onus on researchers to analogize where health care's safety culture has transformed, and uses the body of recent literature to support the assertion. Plenty of literature exists to support the notion that health care's safety culture is transforming (Leape et al., 2009; Wachter,

2010). It must remain only an interpretation—the meaning of text is negotiated in the community of interpreters. A research question could be used to resolve the tension: *where is health care on the continuum of safety culture transformation, in part, through use of aviation-based teamwork methods?"*

I highlight this key conclusion to inform you that the entire point of the book is just my own interpretation. Many other researchers have opinions, too, about these matters. I have carefully given you citations where their work has influenced my efforts, so, if you want, you can read their assertions for yourself and compare my ideas with your own. This rigorous research process is the reasonable way we can collectively work as scholars and practitioners toward culture transformation.

Let me put this into different, perhaps more practical terms. If you hold an evidence-based research mindset, I have included this chapter to serve as a bridge from the lens of aviation teamwork methods, to practical fieldwork in health care settings.

Seeking "Aha" Moments

Another way to view my constructivist perspective is to view learning through a generative development perspective—a series of "light bulbs." I came to a *Befindlichkeit* where I described them as "Aha" moments. When viewed in a continuum, these "Aha" moments form a new way of learning. Included in them is consideration of the notion of didactic, or teaching and observation alignment; to assess other's frustrations or joys in a manner congruent with exploring transformation as a continuum of lived experience.

In case you've been struggling to wrap your arms around ontology and phenomenology, what I just said about "Aha" moments captures the essence. Conroy (2008) described aspects of what I'm providing as "hermeneutic turns" in a study. I entered the continuum of health care's safety culture transformation with a goal of better understanding how far the safety culture has moved with a before to after snapshot of the given experience. Judging better or worse isn't necessarily the goal. I wanted to take a snapshot in time of where health care's safety culture transformation is now, analogous to the 1979 NASA workshop for aviation and the 1999 IOM report.

I discovered an inherent dichotomy with health care research perspectives, and sensed the associated frustration. In doing so, I experienced yet another "Aha" moment. The dichotomy itself produces a healthy tension that perpetuates moving ahead. Many could become discouraged and tired, resulting in complacency and apathy. As I struggled with the process, I endeavored to create rigor and quality for my study, the dissertation manuscript, and this book.

Going back to the core matters themselves is not only important, it is *vital*. It creates a *Befindlichkeit*—an overall essence of learning and discovery, making the encounter worth the time and energy invested.

The Impetus for Organizational Transformation

Experience an encounter like this for yourself. Provide your own opportunity for an "Aha" moment.

When you do you will produce the fulfillment of a lesson learned. The process yields power of heart and passion of existence to achieve error mitigation in individuals and organizations. The cumulative effect provides the impetus for transformation.

Inspiring Distinction, Serving Others, and Building Community: Values Forming the Vision of Teamworks

Inspiring distinction, serving others, and building community comprise the core values to form the vision for **Teamworks**. Perhaps it is more possible now to see the underlying manner in how they were crafted.

Consider this: aviation's teamwork model produces a distinct essence of expertise and precision. When I view the concept, I think of the exacting work of the Navy's TOPGUN school, or four years of training for participating in the Olympic Game race relays, or years of experience on Daytona 500 pit crews to reduce microseconds off a driver's stop time—the difference to win a checkered flag or allow another team to seize the prize.

What does it take for someone to become that good? More than mere knowledge... distinction needs fire, determination, resolve. It's not just what you do. It's who you become. It's who you are.

Addressing these theoretical milestones has been humbling but exhilarating for me. Although I like to think I can become part of a distinct group of practitioners who seek ways to help others overcome their error-prone ways, I come back to the humility of realization that I'm a human, too. I can never forget this. I must always seek to serve others. As I transform my own behavior, I can share lessons of humility that might inspire others. This builds community.

As I conclude this summary of these hallmarks of learning, I invite you to examine my mind-maps at the end of the book that illustrate my research strategy. This examination might help those who want to consider interpretive phenomenology as a way to explore other research problems.

With this review of my theoretical *Befindlichkeit* completed, let's explore what health care respondents had to say about aviation teamwork to mitigate errors. I believe you will find their comments informative and surprising.

> The process yields power of heart and passion of existence to achieve error mitigation in individuals and organizations, to inspire a community, a generation. The cumulative effect provides the impetus for transformation.

Chapter Eight

Real-Life Excerpts from

Health Care Providers

My teenager becomes frustrated when his math teachers ask to see his work when solving problems; sometimes it costs points on exams.

He says, "I gave the correct answer!"

We tell him it's not only the answer that's important; it's how you arrived there.

This chapter is for those who want to see the work, to see "how I arrived there." I encourage you to join me in the spiral of understanding, to search for those small golden nuggets from what others have given us. Some of the passages are long; however, I am convinced of their learning value.

Concluding that health care professionals all want to improve care, think of patients as you read. Indeed our focus is not on just what we learn; it is primarily on how we apply what we learn to affect positive change and cultural transformation.

If you're like me, you believe strongly in doing no harm. Perhaps learning about what others have experienced may help you avoid doing something harmful yourself. In this collection you might find a personal *Befindlichkeit* to offer in the community of learning. Let's see.

Data Statistics and Distillation Steps

Let me give you some details regarding the data I collected and how I distilled it. I transcribed 10 hours and 20 minutes of audio-taped interviews from 10 respondents into a separate document after each session. This took approximately one hour per 10 minutes of recorded time. The transcripts resulted in a total of 85,958 words and 171 single-spaced pages of textual data. The data were distilled into 330 significant statements used to produce 99 meanings, an average of 10 per respondent.

Each transcript was printed and filed into a large binder of data. Transcripts were reviewed manually and significant meanings identified on the left margin with written notes. Colored highlighting markers and marker tapes were used to identify and segregate themes based on participant learning or application of aviation teamwork. A chronological table and mind-map was created for each respondent interview based on the written notes and colored highlights.

During subsequent reviews, major quotes and emergent interview meanings were marked, and additional notes annotated on the right margin in contrasting colors. In the first review, significant meanings were identified in respondents' own words for creation of a chronological table. Connected to "aha" moments, particular attention was given for embedded meanings and trigger phrases such as, "it was funny," "I didn't realize," "a light bulb came on," and so forth to capture emergent vivid lived experiences and identify potential ontological significance.

Learning from the Data

In studying the discourse of transparent data this group of respondents contributed, we have an opportunity to learn. In doing so, we may solidify our convictions about working forward as empowered participants in health care's safety culture transformation.

Let's face it—we all have similar stories, whether they have been told yet or not. Some of these stories you see below may remind you of an experience of your own; but the point is that every observation contributes another opportunity to learn.

My observations are made within quotes by use of brackets [for example]. I have organized the excerpts into four segments.

The first segment addresses thematic clusters I found regarding how health care providers learn teamwork. The second segment addresses clusters of themes regarding how teamwork is used for error mitigation. The third segment addresses emergent themes that I found after adaptation through interpretive phenomenology. I think of them as bonus themes. The fourth segment, a collection of stories that moved me the most, is a series of vivid, real-life error accounts.

The names and organizations are carefully de-identified. We look at these responses not to criticize individuals, departments, or organizations; rather, to look introspectively at how experiences have happened in our own house.

Now, I'm going to get out of the way and let you dig in. Real-life data is presented in indented format for ease in identifying.

First Segment: How Do Health Care Personnel Describe Their Experiences with Learning Aviation Teamwork Methods?

Two areas emerged: implicit learning and real-time learning.
- Implicit learning happens on its own, without being planned or delivered
- Real-time learning, in simple terms—is on the job.

Implicit Learning

All ten (100%) respondents described the implicit manner in which physicians, nurses, and managers learn teamwork.

In the first quote, a participant provided a trigger phrase example:

> "It's funny; I didn't consciously learn it I don't think... I don't remember anyone ever sitting down with me and saying, 'Okay, you're part of a team, and this is how a team works.' I experienced it. When I was an intern, I had a number of different chief residents, and I saw a number of different styles of leadership. I had been a crew chief on an ambulance in college, and saw something similar, but even then, I don't necessarily think that there was anything in particular. I certainly didn't take any courses or read any books that said 'this is how you do it.'" (Respondent H, personal communication, November 11, 2011)

Another participant described the progressive nature of health care learning:

"Who I am today is from studying how others operated and how they have acted in times of stress, during periods where perhaps errors were made, and where members of the team made errors. You remember those cases very well, and it changes the way you practice. Over the years you hone that further as you gain more experience. It's a very interesting progression; it certainly doesn't happen overnight." (Respondent A, personal communication, August 30, 2011)

A third participant commented:

"Certain players that are younger don't see the big picture yet, and they may hinder the process with their lack of experience; they're hyper-focused on their one part. When they're barking out their one part they don't recognize it's not relevant—that nurse can't give me what I'm looking for because they're doing something more important... It's a learning process." (Participant E, personal communication, September 23, 2011)

Yet another participant described physician residents' learning progression:

"One of the major goals of internship is to learn how to acquire data accurately and efficiently; you're not expected to do a lot with the data. Today, there are lots of interns running around gathering notes... As a mid-level you take that data and do something with it, interpret it, develop treatment plans; you don't have to spend time and energy getting the data for making a decision—you've learned how to do that already... It's not formalized, but there's no question the chief resident makes sure the entire team is working together to cover the floor." (Respondent H, personal communication, November 11, 2011)

A fifth participant described the inferred, ad hoc nature of health care education:

> "In terms of actual teaching of these things [teamwork, checklists, briefings] it's been very ad hoc. Was a demonstration, very little in the way of actual; certainly nothing in the way of didactic teaching about how teams should operate. I happen to believe in teamwork, but have no idea how to teach it at a didactic level." (Respondent B, personal communication, August 30, 2011)

Further, a participant discussed an experience in an emergency room setting:

> "You put these pads on him, then you can hands-off shock him; and so, somebody said, 'So let's put him on the pads." A new nurse was standing there looking at the defibrillator that we have, and I'm watching her, right...

and I say, 'You gonna do that?' And she says, 'Well, yeah." I go, 'Do you know how to use that?' And she goes, 'Well, I'm signed off.' I said, 'But have you ever done it, have you ever touched one before?' She goes, 'No. Once you're signed off on something, you're signed off for life.'" (Respondent C, personal communication, August 31, 2011)

Another respondent described vivid thoughts of learning CRM as a flight nurse and related it to the current nursing setting (an additional trigger phrase example):

"I never really thought about this until now, you learn the CRM and you learn the pieces of it. It all has relevance in multiple venues of our life, but we don't learn it in the same fashion with those pieces. I think it would be helpful to learn it with all of those pieces, and say, this is how it applies, this is how this (emphasis) applies to your world, this is how this (emphasis) piece applies to your world... [Yes, it's repeated twice] - I think that would be different in each department perhaps and in each setting, but I think it would be valuable to do that. To assimilate it with examples in each world so you could understand how each of the pieces fit. We learn it, but it's kind of fragmented though; where we say okay, it's important to have communication between each of the caregivers and it's important to read back orders and it's important to go through this checklist when you do this procedure. But it's fragmented into different pieces and parts. There's not global learning, like, this is CRM and here are the pieces, and here's how it applies to your world. It just doesn't box that way; it may be easier for people to learn if it was that way." (Respondent D, personal communication, September 19, 2011)

While discussing assertiveness, a participant recalled an experience during residency where nurses "hijacked" the situation:

> "The team leader may not be able to step up and lead, and be confident. Senior nursing staff may actually hijack a lower-level resident; it falls back on the loudest voice. I didn't want a specific medication given and it was given anyway because the nursing staff was so aggressive, and that's what they always did. You can get run over if you are not a strong enough leader. I had to pick it up over time; I'm not being assertive enough. In medical school you're not taking classes with nursing. I think everybody tries to figure it [teamwork, communication, leadership] out." (Respondent F, personal communication, October 27, 2011)

Another participant discussed how staff works together:

> "So less adapted nurses have been treated badly by residents and physicians, so it becomes a pattern to treat residents and physicians badly, even when somebody is being nice to them. I think that is learned—not very helpful." (Respondent B, personal communication, August 30, 2011)

Finally, a participant discussed how staff modeled teamwork:

> "In undergraduate school I saw teamwork modeled... You could recognize, maybe I couldn't define it per se... Because it was just what they happened to do... But you could tell teams that were much more effective... We sub-consciously recognized things about teams... It just happened, it wasn't deliberate. You could see the times where providers

purposefully paid attention to nurses—asked their thoughts and opinions, would read the progress notes, would ask questions... And there were times when some providers who were just [pause]—well, difficult, to say the least. Don't call me. And so you would notice the outcomes." (Respondent I, personal communication, November 28, 2011)

Real-time Learning

Eight respondents (80%) highlighted the presence of real-time, on the spot, on the floor, at the bedside and peer-level learning for health care staff. A participant explained how nurses learn in real-time:

"Sometimes nurses learn better from a peer level rather than an administrative level, because it's a downward force of learning. We're really trying to push with our staff—peer to peer, real time—is always better. If you can take care of it on the spot in real time, and say it would be really good if you did this, it would be better for the patient if you did this." (Respondent D, personal communication, September 19, 2011)

During a follow up question, the same respondent expounded further:

"I think nurses learn at the bedside better than they learn by reading something later. So if they have the ability at the bedside for someone to point out something or even hold them accountable... in real-time when they're doing their job, I think that is a more productive learning environment than sitting in a classroom or reading an e-mail." (Respondent D, personal communication, September 19, 2011)

Another respondent noted the importance of timely communications:

> "If you don't feel open about sharing, things don't get passed on or communicated... There's a missed opportunity to intervene on the spot." (Respondent I, personal communication, November 28, 2011)

While discussing mentoring efforts, the same participant highlighted the importance of sustainment:

> "With planned programs where you have those mentor-preceptors, you carefully select those mentors and then you educate and train, and continually update and sustain that type of program. Then your chances of mentoring those new graduates or any new nurse that comes into your organization... a better chance of assuming or assimilating the values of the institution, the mission, goals, how that

particular unit they may be in… or section, or service operates or works together. I think that's an ideal [emphasis] situation for learning teamwork." (Respondent I, personal communi-cation, November 28, 2011)

A participant noted the use of real-time discussions with videoconference technology:

"We've been pushing technology this year, these are great tools because we would do a lot more real-time face-to-face communication if it were easier to use. We're also doing more with tele-medicine and real-time, face-to-face kinds of things with distances." (Respondent J, personal communication, December 2, 2011)

Yet another participant highlighted the importance of anecdotes and real-life cases:

"The best way to teach other physicians is by anecdote; there's also evidence-based medicine, where research studies come to a conclusion. Those are not as powerful as anecdotes, because physicians remember certain cases... There's nothing like a real-life case to really hit something home. You can talk about 'what if's,' but if you have a real-life case, and this is what happens, you can't argue about that." (Respondent A, personal communication, August 30, 2011)

To summarize the answer to the first research question, learning aspects of health care's safety culture transformation include an implicit learning style and importance of real-time learning for lasting effect. Teamwork learning within health care's safety transformation framework is marked by frustrations among staff and leadership. Learning experiences among respondents reflected a lack of deliberate training regarding teamwork.

Second Segment: How Do Health Care Personnel Describe Their Experiences Applying Aviation Teamwork Methods in Health Care Settings to Mitigate Root Causes of Medical Errors?

Two areas are covered in these responses: structure and the influence of egos.

- Structure is the organizational framework in which staff works.
- Influence of egos is when senior staff members don't listen, or even worse, disparage, insult, or blame teammates.

Structure

All 10 respondents (100%) in the sample discussed application of teamwork in the context of structure, guidelines, process, systems, outcomes, and practice. One participant discussed two noteworthy milestones in health care in the past two decades:

> "The most influential piece in performance improvement over the last 15 or 20 years besides fixing the blame culture was flow mapping; historically, we would just try to go in a room and talk through something, we never put anything on paper... Trying to understand that there are variations on the different ways that people do it... and it's not a standard process... and it was just hit or miss." (Respondent J, personal communication, December 2, 2011)

Another participant compared differences in flexible guidelines to aviation checklists:

> "The physician, who is ultimately responsible for medical management, has the ability to use clinical decision making to veer from those guidelines as they see fit for a situation... In aviation you use the checklist to start the aircraft every single time, but in

medicine it's not as black and white; even though people present the same complaint or have the same diagnosis." (Respondent D, personal communication, September 19, 2011)

Another participant described the wedge between nurses and physicians as a result of implementation of a new medical record system:

> "Now we're completely physically apart; the glass barrier creates a new dynamic of separation between nursing and medicine... Doctors write their orders in a computer; physical findings and patient assessment is discussed without nursing involved. Before they were within earshot, if anything was off you could chime in... Now, there's no collaboration—all medicine in assessment, barfing out the orders for the nurse to complete." (Respondent E, personal communication, September 23, 2011)

Yet another respondent compared health care's response to errors with aviation:

> "We don't do nearly as good a job as aviation does of certainly recording its errors. We do a reasonable job when there has been a bad outcome. We do a terrible job for near misses, and a REALLY terrible job for system issues." (Respondent B, personal communication, August 30, 2011)

A respondent described error reduction efforts to improve outcomes:

> "We are focusing on reducing errors in all aspects of care, including medication errors and administration. Making sure we got the right patient, right drug, right time, and all of those things to reduce any negative outcomes. We put in place procedures specifically associated with reducing those errors: double

checks, checklists, documentation requirements to ensure that those things don't end up occurring... Industry-related items like six sigma and lean processing are being used heavily." (Respondent G, personal communication, November 9, 2011)

Finally, a respondent compared the art of health care practice with aviation:

"So rote, understanding, application, correlation [learning levels taught to flight instructors]—you've been flying for 20 years and above those levels is the art of flying. The doctors start off with the art somewhere between rote and understanding... Only 10% really are effective at the higher level; some of them are using the artistic practice as a crutch... It covers them if they make the wrong decision." (Respondent C, personal communication, August 31, 2011)

Influence of Egos

Seven of 10 respondents (70%) noted the influence of egos upon teamwork application. Three rich illustrative examples follow, beginning with a story about emergency medicine physicians intubating a patient.

> My attending was there with me... He had two very experienced people, who'd done probably 500 intubations in the last few years, and he didn't even ask us—instead he did a surgical cricothyrotomy [cut air hole in patient's windpipe at throat—it leaves nasty scar]. If he couldn't have gotten that airway then it could have gone bad—you're really sunk. So just the hubris of that moment has always stuck with me, to try and be able to stand back and not have your ego get too much in the way of decisions you're making. (Respondent B, personal communication, August 30, 2011)

Another participant highlighted adverse impacts of egos while serving as a non-profit volunteer in Russia and compared this experience to applied teamwork in the United States:

> "The doctors in Russia, they don't like having other people question them—this is a huge obstacle to overcome... They don't understand the elements of teamwork that are necessary to do these operations and to have their kids do well... So helping them to get to understand the importance of teamwork is really key, and doing similar things—the checklist, and communication needs to occur and getting to the point, sometimes, where look, this is a critical team member who's not able to do the job because they're stubborn or because they're unwilling for whatever reason... Look they've got to go, they can't be part of the team, if that's the attitude... This isn't personal, this isn't about ego; it's about

what your goal is. We've travelled all these miles and it's not going to be pleasant at times. You're going to have to change the way you do things." (Respondent H, personal communication, November 11, 2011)

Finally, a respondent discussed how some staff disregarded safety policy:

"You have a process, it's been vetted through multiple stages and fine-tuning and then you have people that just don't want to do those safety checks. They don't want to scan the armbands—they want to do work arounds. They don't want to do an identification of the patient using the identifiers; they do work arounds where they blatantly disregard that." (Respondent J, personal communication, December 2, 2011)

Third Segment: Bonus Themes

During entry into the hermeneutic circle, I subjected the respondent's data to adaptation through interpretive phenomenology. As I conducted the research, a number of additional items emerged, outside the scope of my initial research design. Think of them as bonus findings. I discovered three distinct emergent themes: transformation, teamwork, and leadership.

Transformation

Health care remains on a course of change, precipitated in part by the IOM study *To Err is Human* (Kohn et al., 1999). All 10 participant (100%) interviews reflect an essence discerned as ongoing transformation in the health care community. The *Befindlichkeit* of transformation observed during interviews is a perspective of struggle, conflict, and division in varying degrees across disciplines and communities moving toward an outlook of hope, improvement, and safety.

All 10 respondents (100%) suggested health care's culture is transforming in the right direction, albeit slowly. A prominent thematic context of health care's transformation includes migration from physician-centric to patient-centric care. A respondent described the phenomenon:

> "In the past, health care delivery has been physician centric; with the physician as the most knowledgeable member of the team— their preference, attitude, and style would drive the team in whichever direction it was going to go. At this point, I think we're moving away from the physician being the most important aspect of the team and their desires, wishes being carried out to really that... The patient and the family being the most important person of the team and they are considered part of the team... And designing systems and processes around what the patient is going to desire." (Respondent G, personal communication, November 9, 2011)

Further, the same respondent explained the struggle of health care's transformation:

> "So, if we're talking about global change that our organization's going to make, you're always going to have those on the side that are in favor and those that aren't. And when I talked about patient-centered versus physician-centered, I think we're still struggling with—how do we get physicians on board for certain aspects of what we're doing?" (Respondent G, personal communication, November 9, 2011)

In a context of early medical school training and resident learning in the 1990s, a respondent noted:

> "Surgeons would be very autocratic and didactic; rigid, authoritarian figures—it was the system; everything revolved around them. The more old-fashioned medical model

will have the nursing staff on a rung lower than physicians. It's, 'I am the top of the pile and you do not question me'; it can be painful and annoying to be constantly questioned by people who have no clue what's going on. I find it very useful to be questioned by people who DO [emphasis added] know what's going on and I think that's one thing aviation has done much better than medicine has." (Respondent B, personal communication, August 30, 2011)

Another participant said:

"[Un-named influential leader] is an intimidating person; you might not know moment to moment the reaction. I think having team training to promote communication between multiple levels in the [department] is not a successful endeavor; now they're going to do it again. When you haven't addressed the root issues, how are you going to have change?" (Respondent I, personal communication, November 28, 2011)

Related aspects of organizational focus shifting from physician-centered to patient-centered care include strong and opinionated personalities, illustrated by another participant account:

> "Someone who wants to come in and be the dictator—it won't work in our system. Our department is filled with individuals who are autonomous and opinionated, they are very strong personalities, and they don't necessarily take well to being told what to do; especially if they have a better way of doing it. So I think aviation management would be difficult to apply per se to what we do, but I think it would be a fantastic goal nonetheless." (Respondent A, personal communication, August 30, 2011)

Another respondent illustrated health care's culture transformation toward increased patient safety, commenting:

> "And now, I think the culture is that we're moving much away from that; more toward a patient safety advocacy. It's doing the right thing for the patient... I think all this came from the *To Err is Human* article and we all sort of see that as a wakeup call to medicine. And that's probably where the divide is—those people that really took that report to heart, to change the system—and those who maybe don't." (Respondent F, personal communication, October 27, 2011)

The same respondent later noted:

> "The best thing for the patient is not one person who knows everything, but that EVERYBODY knows it. You have to work in

conjunction with the team—you as a doctor can't know everything and to understand that and understand that you need the knowledge and experience of the nurses, you need the knowledge and experience of the respiratory therapists—you need an entire team to take care of a patient, not just a doctor." (Respondent F, personal communication, October 27, 2011)

Teamwork

Health care teamwork, as perceived, occurs at the grass roots level, from the bottom-up. The *Befindlichkeit* of desired health care teamwork is an essence of special core groups of experts who in many cases work together all the time. Physicians, nurses, and ancillary staff share obligation to one another in a committed sense of community, resulting in higher productivity, effectiveness, and cohesion. Staff members use transparent communications with each other and their patients in a climate free of fear or blame.

The resulting closeness and trust among personnel resonates with synergistic energy.

> The *Befindlichkeit* of desired health care teamwork is an essence of special core groups of experts who in many cases work together all the time.

During participant interviews, I discerned three distinct examples within health care teams to affect improved patient outcomes. The first example was noted as respondents discussed prior experience with emergency medical services (EMS) helicopter operations. Participants compared teamwork in existing health care settings through a lens of their own conceptual experiences with EMS. During interviews, salient areas were probed; respondent comments illustrate a Heideggerian 'clearing in the woods' as described by Conroy (2003):

"Although I was a flight nurse, it wasn't apparent to me aviation teamwork can transition to medical applicability... I wouldn't even have thought of it if I hadn't have talked to you, but we pick out those pieces, and we talk about communication and being assertive and situational awareness. We talk about those things but we don't talk about them in a systems (emphasis) perspective where it could be very much applicable to say this is our crew resource management goal. We're going to focus on each of these individual pieces and this is how we are going to do it. But we've never done that... We don't put it together in a formal manner and I don't know why—especially since I have that background [EMS]." (Respondent D, personal communication, September 19, 2011)

Another respondent compared EMS teamwork with the current health care setting:

"One nurse came from downstairs—'...It's like you guys [small group of former EMS nurses] have this thing (emphasis) that no one else has... There's something that you guys have that I'll never have.' And I thought, 'Ah, wow—that is probably true.' She's a great nurse and a great person, and she works well in a team—but I thought that was kind of interesting that she pointed that out." (Respondent E, personal communication, September 23, 2011)

The next example emerged during an interview with a participant describing a collective effort of the night shift learning how to brief physicians late at night. The charge nurse mentored junior staff to collect patient details prior to briefing harried physicians during the graveyard shift.

Over time, both nurses and physicians noted teamwork synergy as a result of proactive communications.

"I've always learned, and it's very important if I'm going to call a provider at 2 o'clock in the morning, that I have as many facts as I can together. I can understand impatience in that call, and you don't get the information to make a sound decision. So I've found that created credibility on my part with those providers, and it increased the exchange and respect. When I was charge nurse of a [unnamed department]... I worked with nurses and assistants, and they asked me to come to a room and assess a patient. Or they would call and want me to call the provider, because I was the only one who could accept orders and they would start giving me feedback and I would ask THEM for information, and they would ask, [hushed voice, meek, inquisitive tone] 'Why are you asking this?' And I would say, "BECAUSE [emphasis, confident tone]... This is information that I have got to say...' so after time that developed their skills as well... And the team, so over time the night shift was recognized by the providers; they would ask, 'Who's going to be on?' And if they knew our particular team was going to be on—they had more trust. They knew that if we called them there was a reason they needed to respond, because we wouldn't be calling them just to wake them up... So over time the nursing assistants as well as the LPNs (Licensed Practical Nurse), if they called me, they would provide that information to me and then there were other questions I could ask them—so by the time I called the provider, a lot of this information we would go ahead and provide—up front—the provider didn't have to pull it from us. So it developed their skills and knowledge base... We were better able to take care of the patient." (Respondent I, personal communication, November 28, 2011)

Another participant affirmed difficulty achieving a sense of teamwork among spread out entities:

> "The communication piece has been challenging for us since we are so spread out… You lose a sense of community and a sense of obligation to one another, you become dehumanized and your productivity and effectiveness reduces." (Respondent J, personal communication, December 2, 2011).

Finally, the third example comes from a participant description of a teamwork model learned at a conference by Dr. Elliott from London's Great Ormond Street Children's Hospital (Catchpole et al., 2007; Duffin, 2006). The respondent noted:

"The culture we have on the team—it's not endemic; it doesn't exist at all levels, but it should. Everyone has a specific role; they have a job to do... If that breaks down anywhere you've got a problem... It's important for everyone on the team to have a good sense of what their other teammates do and when they do it and how it overlaps... It's important to communicate that to help each other... I also think it's important to understand when it's appropriate NOT to communicate... It really makes a difference in patient care when the nurses, anesthesiologists, and physicians give a very formalized sign out—like a checklist." (Respondent H, personal communication, November 11, 2011)

The same respondent outlined characteristics of effective teamwork:

1. "Core group is together for 4-5 years
2. Specialized equipment expertise

3. Checklists
4. Briefings
5. Situational awareness
6. Precise communications—few extraneous words
7. Climate of expertise and professionalism." (Respondent H, personal communication, November 11, 2011)

To achieve effective teamwork, the participant described action steps:
1. "Awareness of case complexities
2. Slow, step-by-step approach
3. Needs to be very collaborative
4. Bring everyone to the table
5. Get buy-in early." (Respondent H, personal communication, November 11, 2011)

Leadership

The *Befindlichkeit* of leadership among participants reflects influence of lean practice to optimize productivity and enhance the financial bottom line. All 10 participants (100%) discussed gaps between line staff and management; a universal essence of busyness is perceived among health care staff to remain aligned. In at least one department, an underlying tone of complacency, interdepartmental rivalry and unhealthy competitiveness was noted, a minority characteristic perceived from two respondents (20%).

In many cases, the type of leadership to achieve desired patient outcomes is bottom-up, similar to teamwork efforts. Perplexity and frustration remains in health care regarding efforts by staff to transform care toward a patient-centered model. When discussing how to advocate aviation teamwork methods, a participant said peers thought he was an elitist, illustrating an ongoing struggle among health care leadership circles regards how to implement teamwork initiatives (Participant H, personal communication, November 11, 2011).

> The *Befindlichkeit* of leadership among participants reflects influence of lean practice to optimize productivity and enhance the financial bottom line…
> In many cases, the type of leadership
> to achieve desired patient outcomes
> is bottom-up, similar to teamwork efforts.

The following rich and insightful example illustrates the essence of all three emergent themes of transformation, teamwork and leadership:

> "People just don't get it! When I was getting buy-in from my leadership, we have a core group of [medical discipline] that takes care of patients. We have the same [staff], and probably 80% of their duty, clinically, is in the [unnamed hospital area]. In order to get that, I

had to convince the head of [unnamed leader] that, 'Look—this isn't about what I want here. This is about getting a group of people who have a passion for these patients. They'll take better care of the patients, they'll think of more innovations. They'll do a better job if they like what they are doing...' [very animated and emotional]... It's pretty basic here." (Participant H, personal communication, November 11, 2011)

Another respondent discussed a leadership alignment problem during a previous assignment at a large hospital [not in the study population]:

"When I got there the Chief of Staff, Chief Nurse, and Chief Medical Officer didn't work well together. They would get up at the conference room table screaming at each other in the presence of staff or walk out of the room—it was dysfunctional... Or block another on moving forward with policy changes or service changes. It had a strong trickle down effect to all services; there were lots of good people, but when your senior leadership does not work well together, you don't fly." (Respondent I, personal communication, November 28, 2011)

Yet another participant noted difficulty with changes due to personalities:

"If you talk individually with somebody they'll realize the need for something like this. But then when you go and try to implement it, as an industry standard or even a hospital standard, there is [sic] basically too many personalities involved and how it will affect them—that limit or dictate what you are going to do with something." (Respondent C, personal communication, August 31, 2011)

This respondent described financial aspects of care when discussing teamwork:

> "Part of that is financially motivated; if you don't get into that 90-minute window [for a STEMI (ST elevation myocardial infarction) alert] then Medicare doesn't pay for that patient... We have a few other clinical situations that work as smooth as an ST element MI... My guess is we don't have that financial motivation and those tend not to go more smoothly." (Respondent F, personal communication, October 27, 2011)

Regarding real time charting practices, a respondent noted the process of error disclosure:

> "When an error happens, disclosing it to the patient is very important. Documenting it, discussing it, and those are things that happen very regularly. We don't try and sweep it

under the rug. There are too many witnesses — it wouldn't work. You can't do it here. You have to be accountable, that's a big deal. Once you learn that you can be accountable, then you can change your charting practice and your documentation; you are very much complete and careful about what you put in there. You keep it based on the facts." (Respondent A, personal communication, August 30, 2011)

Another participant described an organization's disclosure policy in a deliberate and detailed manner:

"We actually won a patient safety award for our disclosure process; pretty much laid it out on the line — what occurred, what we did to prevent it, what we're doing to prevent it from happening again… It reduces legalities, lowers tort claims and court cases… Also mitigates staff guilt and remorse." (Respondent J, personal communication, December 2, 2011)

Note how this respondent talked about busyness and leadership in the context of education:

"Everyone has their own thing and their own agenda and we don't unify… You know, we've spent the last eight, ten years of our lives getting to the point where we know what we're doing, and we don't need more education just to learn how to do teamwork. We feel (emphasis) that we should know how to do that as physicians. I'm not sure nursing feels the same way… But everybody's tired. And the more sort of regulation that's out there, people become even more tired… It's just fatigue, people don't want to do the extra training to learn how to do teamwork when they have all this other training that they have to do." (Respondent F, personal communication, October 27, 2011)

Finally, another respondent described leadership gaps:

"No one feels like a leader anymore; it's causing problems with getting change to occur; confusion with authority and roles... We have lots of teams coming together recommending change, but no strong leaders taking action to put recommendations into play; we've delegated responsibilities. We do process transformation well but we're not doing well with 'Leadership 101.'" (Respondent J, personal communication, December 2, 2011)

Fourth Segment: Vivid Real-Life Error Accounts

During fieldwork, I was amazed at the integrity and courage displayed by many who recounted memorable experiences of real-life errors. These instances actually happened; the stories are unedited. I certify that I transcribed them verbatim from my audio device used during interviews. The first illustration involves a medication error affecting a little boy:

> "The drug came in a vial, we had a box of the drug I was supposed to give, and a similar drug was OUT of the box but lay up against it... When you look at it, you say, 'Well, okay, that's the last one out of that box.' So I got it, and the procedure was to draw the medication, have it checked by another staff member, which I did, then gave the drug. The little boy was sleepy for a long period of time, and we were trying to figure out why... We sent him home, and at the end of the shift we were required to count the drugs, and we were counting, and we're over on one and under on another and it dawned on me what happened. We had to call them back in. I felt so bad I was shaking—the emotion was so overwhelming;

that I might have hurt this patient. So eventually you regain your composure, and I went in and apologized to the family member; who said, 'It must have taken a lot for you to come in here and say that to me. It's no big deal—he's fine.'" (Participant C, personal communication, August 31, 2011)

Another participant described a story with a similar situation:

> "I popped the top and drew up the med. I looked at the bottle, and it wasn't what I wanted. So it was atropine, instead of this other med that's very similar in size, but completely different, glycopyrolate—and if I hadn't looked at the bottle, and thought, 'These caps are slightly different...' It wouldn't have been life threatening, but it's NOT [emphasis added] the right medication. So, I pull all of them out, and lay them all out and well, half

of them were atropine and half glycopyrolate in the same place. So pharmacy put the two meds in one thing because they look alike; I wrote an incident report that I almost gave the wrong medication because they were in the same compartment and then my manager came in the next day and hugged me... I want everyone to know that glycopyrolate looks like atropine, so no one else does what I almost did." (Respondent E, personal communication, September 23, 2011)

Yet another participant discussed a dose error:

"A patient came in who had taken an overdose of certain medications and was extremely sick... The way you resuscitate them is to give a lot of one certain drug, which was done, and the patient improved significantly to stable... But the drip wasn't turned off and that certain drug kept being given. And so the thing that saved them ended up killing them... a very long and painful death afterwards... Basically the drip was needed for an hour, maybe ninety minutes and it ran for six hours. To wonder if you were directly responsible... It's pretty awful." (Respondent B, personal communication, August 30, 2011)

Another respondent noted a teamwork lapse associated with equipment malfunction:

"I'll give you a classic example for assertiveness, when communication broke down. Had a patient enter heart surgery, was not doing well, need to stay on the heart-lung machine to rest the heart. That type of heart-lung machine is called ECMO. So, I'm busy with bleeding in the chest, totally lost situational awareness because I'm focusing on bleeding during that time. Anesthesia notices that the blood pressure is low.

Perfusion is looking at their flow. Everyone has lost situational awareness now. Luckily my assistant didn't, who looks up and says blood pressure's low. And I look up and say to anesthesia, 'What's going on?' And I say to perfusion, 'What's going on?' So this whole time we're still bleeding a lot, so I have to deal with that. And I hear from perfusion, well, we're flowing, enough, and anesthesia says, 'Well, if you're flowing enough then the blood pressure shouldn't be low because we're giving medicine for that.' So, I tell the assistant, 'I need to deal with this. You deal with the perfusion and blood pressure, anesthesia issue while I deal with this.' Which is what happened, and it turned out, actually there was a flow probe that had malfunctioned. We debriefed... If my head's in the sand, someone else has got to be able to say, 'Hey, we need to fix this problem...' Now what happens is a lot more communication between anesthesia and perfusion while we're on bypass." (Respondent H, personal communication, November 11, 2011)

Yet another equipment-related situation:

"One of the colonoscopes had not been properly reprocessed, and as a result many people ended up with different types of infections or infectious diseases... So they're supposed to do the gross contamination piece before the equipment goes to the central decontamination area; which is kind of huge, because the providers don't want to do competencies... It's been a big hurdle for everyone involved in trying to clean up our processes with that and become standardized." (Respondent J, personal communication, December 2, 2011)

Another surgical case in which a respondent discussed a missed intervention opportunity due to lack of assertiveness:

> "You notice that the secretions coming out of a nasal gastric tube are decreased, and well, okay, you know, that's okay, but maybe it isn't because the previous hour there was half a quart of fluid coming out—and you notice it, and you've irrigated it, but you notice it's changed but, you know, that provider isn't going to pay attention to me anyway, I'm just not going to pass that [information about change] on… You know, they'll see it in intake and output. Well, it could be that the nasal gastric tube is dislodged, so here we go, and then the patient's abdomen is distended." (Respondent I, personal communication, November 28, 2011)

Lastly, a participant recounted a heart patient case with intense and rich detail:

"I remember a patient with a terrible cardiac arrhythmia—her heart was beating very slowly, and was about to stop. And I was like, well, we need to put a pacemaker in her... We need to do this right now. So what that involves is we need to put a central line inside her internal jugular vein, so we set about doing that, and I let the senior resident do it. It's not a junior resident procedure. It's the senior resident. 'We got to do it now,' told her, 'We needed to do this,' she said, 'Okay.' We didn't have time to get written consent, didn't have time to talk about all the risks and whatever—this was kind of a do or die procedure. So the senior resident tried to do it, but he couldn't get the needle into the internal jugular. He tried, and tried, and finally said, 'I can't do it. You got to step in here and do it.' I said, 'No, [strong emotion and emphasis] I want you to step back for a moment, then try again.' Well, he did, and couldn't do it. And he again said, 'I can't do it, please... Will you take this over?' And so, I said, 'Okay,' I stepped in. And everyone was looking at me, so I ended up putting the needle in, I got a flash of blood, and it was bright red, like it was in the vein, I took the wire out, the blood was kind of running out, it wasn't shooting out like it was a jet, like it was arterial, and I said, 'I think we're in' and went ahead and placed the line. And then I realized that it was a fairly brisk return, her pressure was not high, and then I realized that I had put this catheter into her carotid artery. So what ended up happening was she had a large amount of bleeding there. Pulled it out, put pressure on, and then we had to figure out some other way of taking care of her. So, I acknowledged my mistake to the residents, everyone in the room. I told her about it right then and there. I said, 'I made a mistake, I think I put this in your artery and not into your vein, and you're going to lose a lot of blood; you are probably going to need a transfusion.' I said, 'I am very sorry, and I'll do whatever I can to make this up to you.' And I visited the patient every day in the ICU with her family, and I said, 'You know, I'm really sorry this happened.' And the residents saw that I did that, and you know I documented everything. And she ended up doing fine; had a good outcome. I remember it, 'cause it was... I was the final one in the process, and I screwed up and everyone was watching me. So I was justifying doing it because, well, I'm not seeing an arterial pulse. It's just trickling out, it's probably a vein, it's good to go, let's go. Let's do it. And then I heard someone say, 'Are you sure?' And I listened to that... It was the resident who couldn't do it who spoke up." (Respondent A, personal communication, August 30, 2011)

I owe a debt of gratitude to the experts who took time out of their busy schedules to engage in my research study. A courageous journey of *Befindlichkeit* led to incredible discovery for us all. I'm hoping the contextual background I have given combined with these vivid accounts will elicit profound introspection.

Put another way... we need to read these stories and then do some soul-searching on what stories *we* need to tell. *Befindlichkeit* starts with *us*.

We're reaching the home stretch. Let's answer the question, "So... now what?"

> *Befindlichkeit* starts with us.

Chapter Nine

Now What?

During the holiday season, a nurse worked a double shift of more than 16 hours to help an understaffed department. "After getting less than 6 hours sleep prior to a third shift," (Denham, 2007, p. 108) the nurse mixed up two identically shaped clear medication bags. The nurse substituted an epidural bag for the antibiotic bag, resulting in the young mother's death. The organization terminated the nurse without severance compensation; the nurse was also prosecuted as a criminal by the state attorney general office (Denham, 2007). Subsequently, patient safety advocates supported the nurse to spark community-wide changes

(Denham, 2007). Program transformation must be accompanied with processes for catharsis by not only patients, but health care staff affected by errors as well (Gallagher et al., 2003).

As educational foundations of error and systems theory transform, processing of guilt in health care staff and strategies for patient disclosure are vital factors (Wong, Saber, Ma, & Roberts, 2009). In a report analyzing error disclosure, physicians reported feared impacts of disclosure, including litigation, lost trust, adverse reputation impacts, loss of peer respect, and lowered confidence (Gallagher et al., 2003). A 1991 study revealed that 76% of physicians had never told a patient about a significant mistake (Gallagher et al., 2003). Another survey in 2002 noted patients were notified of errors by health professionals only 30% of the time (Blendon, DesRochies, & Brodie, 2002).

Based on my research, I believe recent transparency initiatives have led more organizations to disclose errors to patients. When health organizations work toward a blame-free culture, another underlying problem may arise; the caregivers who commit errors become a second victim (Denham, 2007). Fischer et al. (2006) noted the ubiquity of errors in the medical community, and they reported on the results of 72 students who responded to a University of Massachusetts Medical School study. Students participated in a semi-structured interview, and learning factors included four major topic areas: "personality; hidden curriculum; event characteristics; and role confusion" (Fischer et al., 2006, p. 420). Physicians working in a system in which errors occurred must process their own feelings of "anguish and sense of culpability for errors" (Gallagher et al, 2003, p. 1006).

If you struggle with an error made, I encourage you not to bury it or hide it—for your own sake, your patient's sake, and your family's. Remember, it's less about the who and more about the what. Perhaps you should go to your patient safety manager, or a trusted colleague, and tell them what's on your mind... what's in your gut. Clearly there could be risks here and you would have to assume them; in fact they would be completely yours to own. The point is that admitting error can often be the first step toward a new level of internal understanding and external positive results. When I own my responsibility, then that is *Befindlichkeit* for me. When you own your responsibility, in a full understanding of the circumstances and risks, this can be a part of your *Befindlichkeit*.

Another emerging response to errors is apologies by organizations. Disclosure of errors by health care staff, accompanied in some cases by a carefully crafted apology coupled with immediate restitution of up to $30,000, is another emerging trend (Gallagher et al., 2003; Pawar, 2007; Roberts, 2007). The apology acknowledges medical errors in a structured manner, explains what happened, shows remorse, and offers restitution (Lazare, 2006). Roberts (2007) noted that error disclosure adversely affects patient confidence; however, a more serious problem is failure to disclose, which wears down trust among patients. Roberts (2007) also asserted that an apology should be carefully planned and executed. A good apology contains four components: "Acknowledgement, explanation, expression of remorse, and reparation" (Roberts, 2007, p. 46). Apologies are not preventative, but an apology provides a transparent remediation tool to compensate for medical errors, contrasted with malpractice settlements that facilitate secrecy (Roberts, 2007).

You might say, "Well, I thought about reporting it, but if I do, I'm going to be punished, ridiculed, maybe even fired. I can't afford to lose my job. My organizational culture is still 'blame and shame.'" Let's address these situations.

Tension of Autonomy, Hierarchy, and Blame

An overriding tension in health care is how to detect, report, measure, and mitigate impacts of medical errors (Leape et al., 2009; Wachter, 2010). Root causes of health care's safety culture flaws include traditions of embedded autonomy and entrenched hierarchies. Fischer et al. (2006) noted an informal hidden curriculum that advocates student silence, despite ethical tendencies to speak up when something goes wrong.

A tradition of individual competence praises medical residents as strong when they work well without supervision (Shojania, Fletcher, & Saint, 2006). Although on the surface this approach appears to grow competent physicians, a root cause perspective elucidates problems with excessive fatigue, high workload, and failure of junior staff "to voice concerns in critical situations" (Shojania et al., 2006, p. 595). Steep hierarchies reveal a culture of unhealthy compliance and deference (Walton, 2006).

The most puzzling discovery I made during my research was this: it seems like health care intentionally builds a notion of autonomy rather than **Teamworks**. While autonomy may be necessary in solo providers, this pedagogy seems counter to the overall goal of patient safety. Why would we want to build a defense mechanism into new practitioners that teaches them NOT to listen to or work in collaboration with others?

During Army flight school, it was a proud day when I received my "solo wings." My instructor had given me enough training, and I built the dexterity to pilot a helicopter on my own. Independence and skill emerge as one develops individual expertise. Obviously, I didn't want to always require a flight instructor to accompany me on each flight.

Ego and autonomy are not all bad. Consider the fortitude necessary to command a helicopter and crew, to launch into a storm at night in order to save people from a sinking vessel. The key, however, is balance between ego and teamwork. The experienced helicopter commander listens to his or her crew throughout the mission in a climate of shared understanding.

Some operational venues require autonomy. Consider single-seat aircraft or outpatient settings with a lone provider. But a fighter pilot and a provider must understand personal limitations. There are times when one must embrace, welcome, or demand assistance instead of exercising autonomy.

The goal of **Teamworks** is to educate people in the requisite understanding of when to ask for help. The supporting cast needs to know when and how to speak up, all in the context of avoiding patient harm.

Aviation trains young Captains to use inclusive communication to welcome, even require, input from juniors. Co-pilots learn assertiveness as a core duty and are held accountable for not speaking up. Deference and excessive professional courtesy is of the past.

Pilots who fly alone rely on mechanics, flight planners, air traffic control, instructors, and mentors. Unhealthy autonomy is manifest when pilots believe advice, input, or assistance from others is unnecessary. Many accidents happen when pilots decide to press ahead into weather or other flight conditions beyond their personal limitations. It takes discipline to rein in one's ego and listen to others.

I think we need to train new providers and staff to communicate assertively in a shared spiral of understanding, in order to mitigate errors before the errors result in adverse consequences. This shared understanding is a living, growing context in emergent and dynamic settings.

Sutker (2008) highlighted health care's tradition of autonomy that leads to poor disclosure, transparency, and communication regarding errors. Spath and Minogue (2008) noted errors in health care caused "fear or embarrassment, peer and patient reaction, and litigation" (p. 1). A tradition of blame stifles double loop learning and prevents the changes required to transform health care's safety culture (Stone et al., 2005; Sutker, 2008). A defensive mindset toward error leads to the doom loop instead of transformational culture change (Argyris, 1991).

Hierarchies remain a significant barrier to culture change in health care (Walton, 2006). For outcomes aligned with culture transformation, hierarchy traditions between physicians and residents must shift from a power relationship in which errors are not reported. Indeed, a "patient centred [sic]" model is sought, abounding with "assertiveness and timely and honest reporting" (Walton, 2006, p. 230).

Health care education scholars have acknowledged the problem with autonomy and hierarchy. Through ontological science, I'm convinced we can help individuals and organizations transform the way they handle errors. Look at what aviation did decades ago.

Evaluation of Findings

To review: I adopted a Heideggerian perspective and interpreted the body of data through a lens comparing health care's safety culture transformation with aviation. In the illustrative examples from among 10 participants, 330 significant statements and 99 meanings, I provided a basis for philosophical comparisons between aviation and health care regarding the perspective, timing, and content of teamwork strategies used for medical error mitigation.

In addressing the first research question: *How Do Health Care Personnel Describe Their Experiences with Learning Aviation Teamwork Methods?* I reported how respondents described teamwork as best in real-time or on the floor. Further exploration noted how anecdotes and lessons from operationally relevant settings and contexts might illustrate salient details and optimize learning impact. My interpretation of respondent data included a clear perception that health care teamwork pedagogy lacks deliberate focus, which results in alignment gaps between management and staff.

The second research question was: *How do health care personnel describe their experiences applying aviation teamwork methods in health care settings to mitigate root causes of medical errors?* Regarding this question, I noted unanimous participant support for a health care exemplar of transparency regarding error disclosure with patients, a safety culture attribute advocated by a robust body of research (Leape et al., 2009; Pawar, 2007; Roberts, 2007). The exemplar: apologies work instead of denial.

The series of error disclosure experiences presented in the findings section affirm to the body of researchers the positive value of increased transparency upon culture transformation. Disclosure initiatives among health care staff produce organizational transparency, which in turn fosters increased community accountability. These points remain in alignment with those assertions made by Salas et al. (2006).

Musson and Helmreich (2004) highlighted advances for aircraft operations which stemmed from reporting and analysis, combined with expert opinion. Incongruence with health care research perspectives adversely affects its transformation framework and inhibits teamwork. Indeed, the division must be resolved for effective employment of teamwork methods for medical error mitigation efforts.

Aviation academic leaders teach teamwork concepts early in pilot education and reinforce the concepts during annual refresher training (Salas et al., 2006). Didactic outcomes seem to occur most often with a structured and deliberate focus, and flight crew training includes anecdotal examples from real-life cases and careful emphasis upon the operational context (Musson & Helmreich, 2004). Based on interpretation of respondent data, I suggest that aviation's safety culture is more developed as compared to health care's safety culture. This assertion aligns with similar observations by Leape et al. (2009) and Musson and Helmreich (2004).

Aviation has yet to achieve complete safety, evidenced by two cases illustrating blatant disregard for policy and complacency. In October 2004, two pilots piloted a commuter airliner on an empty leg and for fun decided to attempt a climb to flight level 410 (41,000 feet); the jet suffered a complete loss of engine power (NTSB, 2007). Another case illustrating complacency occurred in January 2009, when an experienced commuter airline Captain failed to monitor and maintain safe airspeed in a snowstorm, resulting in aerodynamic stall (NTSB, 2011). These two cases, among others, have led to NTSB's recommendation and Congress initiating the U.S. Airline Safety and Federal

Aviation Administration Extension Act (2010), which advocates pilot leadership training for the commercial airlines and extends new pilot experience policies for the scheduled airlines.

Comparison with Other Studies

Let's go back to the Space Shuttle *Challenger* example from double loop learning philosophy. Remember that Argyris (1991) described the *Challenger* incident as the doom loop. Staff and management misalignment contributed as a root cause of the catastrophic explosion (Carroll et al., 2006).

Now, compare this example to our examination of health care settings. With the examples from the last chapter, and your own experience, think about it.

Lingering traditions of autonomy and independence create ontology of ego-driven behavior which breeds opportunities for medical errors. Health care staff misalignment with management results in a sense of embedded busyness, which in turn stifles morale and marginalizes safety efforts.

When I debriefed with respondents, showing them this finding, they unanimously told me, "Yes, that's correct." "We want to transform, to improve. But in some regard, we're just stuck."

Do you agree?

> Lingering traditions of autonomy and independence create ontology of ego-driven behavior which breeds opportunities for medical errors. Health care staff misalignment with management results in a sense of embedded busyness, which in turn stifles morale and marginalizes safety efforts.

Leape et al., (2009) discussed transparency gaps with sharing information across health care communities and organizations. Data collected from participants in the present study aligns with this assertion. In aviation, when an urgent safety matter is found on a particular airframe or within a given operational practice, the FAA and NTSB quickly disseminate information to interested parties for rapid action. This practice was not noticed among health care participants in the present study, although one respondent interview noted an organization's establishment of an external peer review program for medical error cases, with experts hired to analyze reports for institutional learning.

Lewis, Vaithianathan, Hockey, Hirst, and Bagian (2011) evaluated and presented a series of 15 steps of safety-related concepts from aviation for use by health care organizations, including a corporate-managed list of minimum standards and a protocol for safety database management. Although aviation achieved a culture of safety among its pilot ranks through CRM and other teamwork methods, learning and application of those methods remains a dynamic transformational process in aviation and other communities.

Salas et al. (2006) noted the importance of a mandate and resources. In 1998, the FAA <u>mandated</u> teamwork training in commercial aviation (Salas et al., 2006). Even though it's not mandatory, do you see the benefit of **Teamworks**?

Effects upon Field of Study

Diverging views abound among health care researchers regarding preferred strategies for patient safety initiatives (Wachter, 2010). Wachter (2010) posited the intuition or anecdotal evidence model, a concept that aligns with participant statements in effective teamwork implementation. In contrast, Wachter (2010) also discussed a tradition of evidence model that aligns with a traditional approach. The pharmacology and disease research communities require randomized controlled studies before embracing change-worthy strategies (Wachter, 2010). Data collected in the present study indicates a need for medical leaders to move on from tradition.

> Data collected in the present study indicates a need for medical leaders to move on from tradition.

It's time for **Teamworks**.

Lerner, Magrane, and Friedman (2009) highlighted a continuing debate in health care regards to timing of introducing teamwork education. The traditional view is to wait until individuals have a professional foundation upon which to offer expertise to a team; however, another view is to start early before attitudes and perspectives become resistant to change (Lerner et al., 2009). Aron and Headrick (2002) noted complete absence of systematic implementation of teamwork training in health care education, but suggested if it were to be implemented, to start early before students become isolated and tainted with a bias of tradition. The larger issue of tradition still requires resolution so health care can agree on timing of teamwork education.

Mohr (2005) highlighted the importance of leadership within health care organizations to foster systemic changes and further discussed double loop learning and technological implementation as two challenges. Mohr (2005) concluded with an impassioned call for further research, affirming the findings of Winokur and Beauregard (2005) who noted leadership and culture transformation as two key elements for improving patient safety. Interpretation of respondent data in the present study matches the observations of Mohr (2005) and Winokur and Beauregard (2005).

> The larger issue of tradition still requires resolution so health care can agree on timing of teamwork education.

Whether it's my style of **Teamworks**, the impressive work of scholar Eduardo Salas, or another program endorsed by The Joint Commission, AHRQ, or IHI, we must recognize the power of working together instead of remaining in silos.

> ...we must recognize the power of working together instead of remaining in silos.

Wachter (2010) lowered the health care community grade for use of technology from B to C, complaining about a downturn in electronic influences upon health care's transformation. Interaction with respondents matches Wachter's (2010) assertions. Further, participant statements about frustrations in electronic medical record (EMR) implementation and a resulting sense of division between medicine and nursing appear an unintended consequence of EMR.

Wells (2007) suggested implementation of evidence-based medicine (EBM) through electronic means would improve patient safety. Wells (2007) research fails to acknowledge health care's divided research, teamwork, and leadership pedagogy. Use of electronic database information in an EBM context within a team environment as suggested by Wells (2007) must include a more developed physical and sociological staff framework prior to effective implementation.

The Wildcard of Generational Differences

While covering the dynamics necessary for cultural transition in health care, I have to mention a wildcard. It's a huge factor and I haven't spent a lot of time on this, but it's another monumental aspect to consider. It is simply this: generational differences. They're present and they're impactful.

These differences can be seen in technology, systems implementation processes, how younger workers expect entitlement early in their career, and how older workers respond with indignation over the notion of paying dues.

To illustrate the phenomenon, I want to share a humorous anecdote from a colleague who wrote it after experiencing the generational differences dynamic in real life.

Mont's Ten Basic Rules for Success in Your New Management Job

1. You're not in college anymore. Dress for success. Think, look, and act sincere. You can horse around on your own time. The boss may inquire politely about your life away from the company, but he or she is just being nice. Your private life isn't rated on the scorecard.

2. Show up for work early. Notice I didn't say "on time." Make the coffee, check your e-mail, clear away your desk for action. Attend all briefings, conference calls, meetings, etc. to which you are invited and take voluminous notes. If you don't need them you can throw them away later. Your boss may ask you to clarify something he or she misunderstood. It's nice to have the correct answer handy. (See Rule 5)

3. Respect the privacy of your peers, superiors and subordinates. Human Resources didn't tell you everything you needed to know before you took this job. It's fair to ask polite questions, but keep them directed toward what you need to know to

accomplish your work. Anything else is invasion of privacy.

4. Keep your eyes and ears mostly open and your mouth mostly shut. Practice the "art of listening." You should be an expert at this after 4 (or 5) years of college. Take a little advice from everyone and use it judiciously. Model after many inputs, not just one. No one person knows everything. Make a list of questions as you read company materials, but don't ask them right away, unless an answer is absolutely necessary in the performance of a job task. See if you can check them off as your weeks progress. It's funny how the answers often show up in routine office conversation.

5. Try to get up on the boards and under the lights with a very few, well-placed shots. In other words, you want early "wins" on tasks you're assigned. The best way to get them is dig, dig, dig. Get the facts, organize your report, coordinate well and do a final edit. Submit your effort on deadline. Don't forget spell checker if you are not an English major.

6. Don't over-worry about what your co-worker is doing, how much they get paid, what your future opportunities are, what the competition is doing, etc. (See rule 3). Opportunities will create themselves only if other people in the company, friends, associates, team members (not just your boss) recognize and comment on your worth.

7. Don't overplay your hand. You may be 23, have a pilot's license and a graduate degree, and think you are God's gift to the company. Maybe. Maybe not. You might be completely surprised to find out you know just enough to get yourself in trouble.

8. If you set to work in a businesslike fashion and accomplish a few early "wins" for which you've received appropriate recognition (like a sincere "thanks" from your boss), you might eventually ask for a consideration—like a few hours off during the workday to handle pressing personal business. Don't push your luck. Remember, there are hundreds of people like you looking to fill just a few available jobs.

9. In almost every job there are issues of great sensitivity, proprietary interest, or what could be called "intellectual property" by the IT types. Learn to regard these issues as you would if you were charged with safeguarding national security. The easiest way to find yourself walking out the door is by betraying a trust or confidence.

10. If most of these rules look absurdly old-fashioned, arcane, or don't jive with your lifestyle, put down your pen and stop filling out the application form. Go home, pour yourself a shooter and call up the old frat gang for a night on the town. Then, after you've called Mommy and Daddy to cry on their shoulder, try to figure out what you are going to do with the rest of your life.

Generational aspects among staff pose a growing portion of leadership's effort to understand key dynamics of health care's safety culture transformation. My study led to a perception that younger workers view technology very differently than older workers. As illustrated by Mont's 10 rules: work ethic, entitlement, and perceptions all play a part.

The issue of generational differences was not considered as part of the problem under exploration in the present study; and therefore was not pursued in depth. While aviation's issue remains automation complacency, health care's implementation of technology appears to create future challenges as momentum builds. Although health care staff has implemented technology, the benefits have not outpaced frustrations over system limitations.

Though not representing a majority finding, two respondents mentioned new divisions between medicine and nursing stemming from recent electronic recordkeeping protocols. Apparently, in the past, they would work together as a team to assess patients and manually write on charts and forms. Now, in one organization's ergonomic design, only a physician sits at a computer screen in an isolated work space, without nursing participation. Nurses still want to be included.

Learning from Past Mistakes

Consider another challenge—the failure to learn from past mistakes. Organizations may have information regarding errors or hazards, but many factors inhibit the flow of data. Implementing a follow-up and follow-through process to pass the word about important information is often forgotten in the reporting-analysis phase. Leaders must emphasize sustainment efforts, including sharing of lessons-learned.

In their management text *Predictable Surprises*, Bazerman and Watkins (2008) described characteristics of organizations that fail to learn from past mistakes:

> "Organizations often fail to learn from past mistakes because they lack the mechanisms needed to share and codify, to the greatest extent possible, key lessons-learned. Such failures may occur because the organization is in a state of overload. Organizations in a

reactive, "firefighting" mode can become trapped in a permanent state of crisis-response that impedes learning. When organizations "patch" serious problems, because they lack the time to identify and correct underlying root causes, the stage is set for predictable surprises." (p. 113-114)

Notice the suggestion to address root causes of underlying organizational learning. We've seen this as a common theme throughout the **Teamworks** model.

With dogged energy and effort we have hope to resolve the organizational learning challenge. Of course, it wouldn't hurt to procure a new electronic system specifically tailored for the purpose and hire a team of eager analysts to assist. In the meantime, maybe a motivated physician or nursing manager could track key items for senior leaders and periodically brief decision makers on progress toward resolution. This would be a good illustration of **Teamworks.**

Summary

These findings herein add to a growing body of data supporting the benefit of aviation teamwork for medical error mitigation (Pratt et al., 2007; Sax et al., 2009). Despite teamwork and leadership gaps, today's health care professionals are ready, willing, and motivated to learn and apply innovative teamwork methods to mitigate medical errors, including methods adapted from the aviation community. As health care leaders recognize a growing trend of collaboration and teamwork toward a model of patient centered care, strong and well-informed leadership must seek to resolve internal and external alignment disparities both in cross-community contexts and within individual organizations.

Taking an aviation program verbatim into a health care setting without specific adaptation, while well intended, may result in more harm than good. Health care community academic leaders advocate an agenda to produce a new generation of collaborative clinicians, in part, through aviation's teamwork model (Kohn et al., 1999; Leape et al., 2009; Lerner et al., 2009; Wachter, 2010).

Here's my conclusion: it's time to combine aviation **Teamworks** with the power of ontology science in health care settings, thereby yielding opportunity for a collective *Befindlichkeit*. Let's not overlook the importance of individual learning combined with informed leadership.

Do we want to continue to suffer negative consequences, or do we care enough to change?

Let's get it done. Let's change our behaviors through **Teamworks.**

Chapter Ten

A Call to Arms

After Nazi Germany invaded Poland, Britain under the leadership of Neville Chamberlain was mired in complacency and confusion. Invited back to the war cabinet only for necessity, Winston Churchill advocated several strategic steps, including mining Germany's Rhine transport artery, cutting off the supply of Swedish iron ore, and seizing Narvik, a key port in Norway. Chamberlain and the majority of the cabinet considered these steps too aggressive. When the Nazis invaded Norway and Denmark the Royal Navy failed to coordinate with the Royal Air Force, and French and British forces suffered thousands of casualties, including the loss of the aircraft carrier HMS Glorious (Downing, 2010). The Chief of Staff, General Sir Edmund Ironside was flabbergasted by the lack of cohesion among his political masters, writing: "Always too late. Changing plans and nobody directing... Very upset at the thought of our incompetence. This was clearly no way to run a war" (Downing, 2010, p. 26).

This is the final chapter. You are invited to process these thoughts and decide on how to respond. Do you have a plan for victory? Or, are you mired with indecision, incompetence, lack of focus?

Enter Teamworks

You can change things. Of this I am fully convinced. Together, we can change things.

One fifth of the United States gross domestic product over the next ten years will be invested in health care (Callendar, Hastings, Hemsley, Morris, & Peregrine, 2007).

Teamworks education must begin early in all health care education venues, and focus toward accountability in the larger team and organizational context rather than placing the entire burden of a flawless patient outcome upon individual providers.

I think this may be the difference between positive, forward-thinking, acting impact and the progression of mediocrity toward health care's safety culture transformation. While individuals working together make a series of small differences, organizations making the bold decisions to transform their culture will make huge differences.

Health care personnel learn teamwork best in real-time, on the floor, with anecdotes and lessons from operationally relevant settings and contexts to illustrate salient details. Current methods for teaching teamwork in health care settings seem to not include a deliberate, focused style. Instead, health care personnel appear to learn teamwork in an implicit or inferred manner. Unfortunately, this tacit method for educating and training health care personnel seems incompatible with a vision for swift-paced safety transformation. Let's change it.

> While individuals working together make a series of small differences, organizations making the bold decisions to transform their culture will make huge differences.

Learning in health care remains influenced by hierarchy and tradition, which in turn produces a flawed perspective of teamwork and leadership by certain people in leadership positions—some physicians. Leadership gaps result when prevailing management philosophies miss their mark. Staff members take matters into their own hands to get the job done. The resulting tension creates a healthy awareness, yet continued struggle leads to frustration and division; symbolized in an inherent dichotomy in health care between advocates of evidence and intuition for safety transformation. Let's change it.

The demands of robust root cause-based systems continue to converge with constrained resources, yielding a need for renewed focus on double loop learning, transparency, and emphasis on a culture of safety. Caretakers of the medical community's academic foundations must emphasize teamwork over independence and adopt blame-free reporting coupled with system improvements to mitigate errors and reduce patient harm (Reason, 2000).

Adherence to the intuition or anecdotal evidence model as suggested by Wachter (2010) aligns with participant statements in effective teamwork implementation. In contrast, a strict tradition of evidence model adheres to the scientific approach aligned with pharmacology and disease research communities, which require randomized controlled studies before embracing change-worthy strategies (Wachter, 2010). Health care learning must continue to transform toward a model aligned with collaboration and teamwork instead of hierarchy and autonomy. Yes, this is where change begins.

If we need to do more studies to evaluate the impacts of **Teamworks** implementations, let's do it. Let's share the results, and collectively move forward. Remember, learning becomes living when behaviors change. **Teamworks** is a method of transferring what we are learning into sustainable results that live.

Bazerman and Watkins (2008) suggested tacit knowledge transfer is difficult to sustain, both individually and in groups. Therefore, health care's safety culture transformation will remain slow without a more deliberate approach to institutionalize, formalize, and standardize teamwork protocols early in physician and nurse training. So, let's start and start early.

In the course of the study, I was surprised to discover that blame appeared not to be a significant concern among respondents. In fact, one respondent confidently stated that a no-blame culture was an organizational norm. Similarly, I expected more respondent input regarding adverse fatigue impacts. Reflected in literature found in the study, reforms in health care seem to align with aviation practices to limit crew time for safety reasons. Absence of a blame culture is a good trend; however, the influence of tradition in teamwork education remains a significant matter for health care educators to resolve. **Teamworks** can help them resolve the issue.

Aviation has experienced similar cases of either blatant disregard or complacency, evidenced by recent implementation of leadership training for pilots in the commercial airlines. Leadership misalignment in health care appears related to opposing philosophical frameworks by which to judge (and therefore pursue) safety transformation efforts. Leadership toward a culture of compliance and discipline remains a significant matter for health care community attention (Leape et al, 2009). **Teamworks** enters here, too, to help leaders and staff align expectations between blameworthy events and "honest mistakes" to resolve them with a systems approach.

Put a different way: instead of asking about whose fault an error was, we need to continue transforming our culture toward asking how to resolve systems issues. We're on the way, but a long journey remains. The exciting part: we all have opportunity to blaze new trails, chart different courses, and file new flight plans.

> The exciting part: we all have opportunity to blaze new trails, chart different courses, and file new flight plans.

Health care lacks central enforcement and investigative entities analogous to the FAA and NTSB in aviation. With health care's indirect, inferred education model for non-clinical topics, leadership is taught the same way as teamwork, producing suboptimal results. Without mandates and resources to produce leadership and accountability, health care efforts to transform toward a culture of safety may remain on its current sluggish trajectory. With a migration in health care toward increased accountability, "no-pay" policies must remain systems versus person oriented. Although outside the study's scope for in-depth review, generational differences affect perceptions toward ontological aspects of teamwork learning and application.

I'm convinced that the best leaders must adopt an ontology lens to view generational differences. The older generation needs to change first; it's essential to initially meet the younger generation where they are.

A New Theory and Its New Behaviors

This book introduces a new theory. It is this: the science of ontology provides powerful learning potential to aid in transforming health care's safety culture.

Think of it as the *Befindlichkeit* approach. How would a richer understanding of *being* influence what you *know* to change what you *do*?

While a growing body of research was discovered citing aviation teamwork for medical error mitigation in health care, limited qualitative studies were present, with none focusing on phenomenological or ontological aspects. A tone of perplexity and frustration abounds in the literature; yet, nobody seemed to offer explanations for root causes of the lack of alignment between staff and management. The data within this study serves to increase understanding within health care's transformational framework ontology.

And this leads us to consider a new way of thinking as individuals and organizations. As we change our thinking, we change what we do. As we change what we do, we change who we are. In changing who we are, we transform our culture.

> Think of it as the *Befindlichkeit* approach. How would a richer understanding of *being* influence what you *know* to change what you *do*?

Teamworks Recommendations

In order to inspire effective teamwork, health care must deliberately teach teamwork early in all of its various school curricula. Health care research initiatives remain affected by stubborn divisions in its academic foundations between process and tradition and with its corporate foundations between profit and people.

Desires for change must begin with decision makers emboldened enough to change their own behaviors. Strong actions may thereby affect transformation for an entire culture.

Medicine needs to heighten focus toward teamwork effectiveness, in balance with individual competence during training.

Recommendations for Practice

As we have learned, health care's art of practice pedagogy produces steep hierarchies (Sutker, 2008). Walton (2006) noted hierarchical effects in producing strong physician egos. These two influences were noted during participant interviews, and appear related to one another as factors stifling health care's safety culture transformation. The essence of participant perspectives in the study reflects motivation for improved health care teamwork, yet efforts remain unfocused, lack coherence, and in many cases are not optimized. Medicine needs to heighten focus toward teamwork effectiveness, in balance with individual competence during training. These two go together.

Aviation began its transformation in the early 1980s and leaders still battle employee disregard and complacency. A new generation of pilots educated in assertiveness and leadership has replaced the older model of power and prestige. Aviation safety culture efforts continue, while targeting increased team leadership, asset recapitalization, and maintenance of aging airframes in today's economic climate of austerity and uncertainty.

Mutual Learning and Living

Indeed, aviation continues work to transform its safety culture, but health care may offer aviation some lessons of its own. For example, Dr. Elliott's consultation with Ferrari race team leaders fostered team communication improvements in a pediatric cardiac surgery clinic (Catchpole et al., 2007).

These collective efforts illustrate cross-community aspects between industries, and in particular could be adapted for aviation maintenance practices to mitigate handover errors. In the spirit of customer service, aviation voluntarily practices policies for refunds or credits for future flights when passengers receive sub-par service (late flight, lost baggage, wrong seat, etc.), analogous to Medicare's no-pay.

In organizations I researched, career nurses ran the quality department. I wondered about the absence of physicians. Let's compare with aviation.

In aviation, experienced pilots serve in an expert role to guide transformation in response to emergent discoveries. It may serve health care organizations well to assign physicians as patient safety researchers in their quality and performance improvement departments. Health care has yielded significant gains in transparency efforts through successful implementation of disclosure policies. The medical community has a new opportunity to build upon these gains in both internal and external health care settings with a new spirit of alignment toward accountability and EMR implementation.

Without national-level governing and investigating entities, analogous to the FAA and NTSB, health care efforts toward safety through teamwork will continue to lack accountability and focus. As postulated by Salas et al. (2006), mandatory implementation combined with sufficient resources are core ingredients for effective teamwork. The efforts of non-mandatory entities in health care such as AHRQ, IHI, and The Leapfrog Group remain commendable, but simply do not achieve the same results as aviation has achieved following implementation of the FAA in 1958 and NTSB in 1966.

Recommendations for Future Research

Research into sociological and ontological transformation among health care practitioners toward patient-centered care remains incomplete. Health care's academic inquiry efforts appear focused upon pharmacology and disease investigation rather than organizational change among staff. Many health care leaders contend with frustration and division regarding teamwork and error mitigation initiatives (Leape et al., 2009; Wachter, 2010). Health care academia *must* investigate consequences of not teaching teamwork early in medical and nursing school curricula; moreover, integrating teamwork education into health care's academic foundations may accelerate the pace toward safety transformation.

Health care remains centrally focused upon impersonal application of lean management to influence staff and enhance corporate profitability. While a profit-motivated approach upon process improvement is perceived as good business, continued endeavors to understand deeply rooted aspects of people issues through qualitative methods will yield dividends. Lingering traditions of hierarchical independence and autonomy among personnel regarding the art of medicine continue to affect pedagogical and research perspectives. These two combined factors (excessive focus upon profits and process over people and clinging to hierarchical tradition) contribute to a leadership gap that inhibits learning and stifles organizational change initiatives.

And let's revisit this one more time: teamwork research in both health care and aviation must include recognition of the growing dynamic of generational differences.

Behavior traits of the middle generation (sometimes known as 'Generation X') and millennial employees include a need for validation and require more robust policy guidance than baby boomers or traditional generation members.

This issue provides researchers another aspect to consider in teamwork and leadership pedagogy, and it should be considered. For effective fielding of electronic technology and integration of systems for more effective processes, increased understanding of generational ontology would be useful.

Alignment and Application

This discourse serves as a catalyst for debate among the research and academic communities in both health care and aviation. Scholars must seek alignment about how and when to educate professionals in collaborative behaviors, including leadership, for operational decision-making. In addition, aviation's academia should note an opportunity to implement practical application of health care best practices, particularly in aviation maintenance processes.

The discussion no longer centers on how aviation teamwork may benefit health care; inherent lessons may transcend from one community to another in a hermeneutical spiral of shared understanding. Phenomenological research exploring health care teamwork applied in aviation settings, using the methods and design herein, would increase credibility, dependability, and transferability of the present study.

The respondents interviewed and overall community of health care leaders seem well aware of gaps between the present and desired attributes of patient care. Unfortunately, many health care personnel do not receive focused education and training regarding teamwork, leadership and collaboration. Health care delivery, including the sociological and ontological aspects of a team-oriented transformation of patient-centered care, remains a top priority.

Reason (1997) eloquently contextualized culture transformation with an ontological perspective: "we must acknowledge the force of the argument asserting that a culture is something that an organization 'is' rather that something it 'has'" (p. 220).

Health care's transformation need not continue at its present sluggish pace. The time is now to recognize the importance of lasting action to resolve long-standing fractures within health care's pedagogical framework to achieve safety culture transformation. In other words, health care needs to come together to decide on the best way to teach and foster **Teamworks** in order to better care for patients.

Ask yourself, "Am I on the same page with my teammates?" Failure to take a deliberate, intentional approach to foster **Teamworks** is a latent, hidden, and subtle flaw. The statistics reveal that safety culture transformation isn't moving as rapidly as most leaders desire. How might a better understanding of *Befindlichkeit* assist these worthy efforts?

The bottom line: we can save lives, decrease injuries, and reduce costs. These are worthwhile goals and their accomplishment is well within our grasp.

Twelve O'clock High

With our World War II theme throughout, I want to draw your attention to a fantastic resource I like to use for safety training. It is the old movie *Twelve O'clock High*, filmed in 1949. You can view it yourself, gather small groups of colleagues or plan a training workshop. My *Transformation Guide* includes a short resource for team facilitators to use while showing the movie.

Your only constraint may be a space large enough to accommodate the group, comfortable seating, and having the video on hand. I purchased my copy of the movie at a bookstore. Be sure to follow all regulations regarding copyright and be sure to secure necessary permissions to show this movie in any venue if required by applicable law.

Remember that showing a film as part of an event for which people have paid an entry or participation fee may constitute a violation of copyright or performance rights. Be sure to check and adhere to the law in all of these matters.

The movie stars Gregory Peck who plays Brigadier General Frank Savage. Savage is a B-17 pilot and Army Air Corps leader. The idea of using *Twelve O'clock High* as a safety and leadership resource has been one of my favorites for many years. In the story you will see a myriad of dynamics, including errors, reporting, and teamwork. You will join the 918th Bomb Group in Archbury, England in mid-1942 as they experience failure, victory, stress, heroism, and valor beyond words. The story continues through months of ups and downs. Supporting actor Dean Jagger won an Academy Award for his brilliant performance as Adjutant Harvey Stovall.

Teamworks

Fire up the popcorn maker. Order pizza. Enjoy.

And let the era of **Teamworks** *begin.*

Acknowledgements

For my wife Elizabeth, sons Cameron, Hunter, and Spencer, and daughter Bethany—you remain inspirations of love, hope, and courage.

I am grateful for the mentoring and guidance from my Dissertation Chair Steve Roussas, Ph.D. and committee members Laura Pogue, D.M. and Doug Mikutel, Ph.D. Also, to Dr. Mike Wetmore, Dr. Steve Munkeby, Dr. Jim Savard and Dr. Kathy Wood for helping me find my way in the doctoral process.

I could not have completed my research without the professional assistance from Dr. Aaron Bair and support from Captain Michael Eagle, U.S. Coast Guard. Vital to credibly pursuing research in health care venues, I'm thankful for the assistance and counsel from Joel Bales, Fellow, American College of Healthcare Executives.

For countless unnamed colleagues and mentors who influenced my aviation leadership philosophy, and faithful Christian colleagues offering generations of encouragement.

Thanks to Glen Aubrey for coaching me to transform my work from an academic to a conversational voice. Also, to Laura Santigian and Keith Berger for their encouragement and insight.

For those who contributed to the foreword and endorsements, I'm grateful. I appreciate the work of Justin Aubrey for the cover, Randy Beck of My Domain Tools (www.mydomaintools.com) for my web design, and Paula Kaplan for my author photo.

Gratitude and love for my parents: Jesse Morrison and Glenda Oetting, and in-laws Carl and Nobuyo Avery.

To God be the glory; all things are through Him.

About the Author

Dr. Mitchell Morrison is a senior Coast Guard officer, an expert safety leader, and distinguished practitioner-scholar in aviation teamwork ontology, having logged over 6,800 pilot hours in various airplanes and helicopters during a career spanning over 30 years.

Along with command cadre and senior management experience, his resume also includes a Ph.D. in Business Administration, Master of Aeronautical Science, Bachelor of Professional Aeronautics, Airline Transport Pilot rating, and Certificate in Aviation Safety. A lifelong learner, Dr. Morrison utilized interpretive phenomenology in his doctoral dissertation research to explore learning and application of aviation teamwork in health care settings for error mitigation. He co-presented a paper on Generational Differences in Aviation Leadership at the 2011 forum of International Society of Air Safety Investigators, and he is published in the proceedings. He taught Operational Risk Management / Aviation Human Factors at the University of California Davis Extension and has ten years of faculty experience with Embry-Riddle Aeronautical University.

Mitch is an avid baseball fan from Little League to the major leagues. He lives in Northern Virginia with his wife and four children.

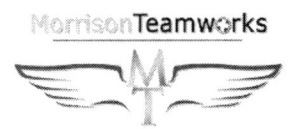

MorrisonTeamworks

www.morrisonteamworks.com

works

www.wxrks.com

Glossary

Definitions

Adverse event: An adverse event is a situation during patient treatment that may or may not result in undesired consequences (Gallagher, Waterman, Ebers, Fraser, & Levinson, 2003; Pratt et al., 2007).

Autonomy: Autonomy is an organizational culture attribute in medicine emphasizing individualism (Sax et al., 2009; Sutker, 2008); performance of expert individual practitioners "trained to be self-sufficient and individually responsible" (Musson & Helmreich, 2004, p. 25); lack of regard for broader team influence (Leonard, Graham, & Bonacum, 2004).

Aviation Teamwork Heuristic: Aviation Teamwork Heuristic (ATH) is an original term created during formation of my dissertation, representing a contextual and interpretive framework characterized by the eureka-like discovery of a dynamic process of shared responsibility, community (e.g., aviation or health care) transformation, learning, and adaptation. Although heuristics are also a form of phenomenology, the intended context of the term ATH is not heuristic inquiry or heuristic research, as described in Shank (2006).

Blameworthy actions: Blameworthy actions are "criminal actions; acts of drug or alcohol abuse during care; actions recognized by individual as unsafe and committed with no mitigating reasons anyway" (Bagian, 2005, p. 8). Marx (2001) established a practical continuum of attitudes and behaviors for health care managers to use while considering blame attribution.

Crew Resource Management (CRM): Introduced in the early 1980s to reduce errors, CRM is effective management of resources by the flight crew, including situational awareness, communications, assertiveness, and risk management (Helmreich, 1996; Weiner, Kanki, & Helmreich, 1993). The Federal Aviation Administration [FAA] (2004) defined CRM as effective use of all available resources, including human, hardware, and information resources.

Culture: Ferguson and Fakelmann (2005) quoted Reason's (1997) definition of culture: "Shared values (what is important) and beliefs (how things work) that interact with the organizations' structures and control systems to produce behavioral norms (the way we do things around here)" (p. 34).

Double Loop Learning: Argyris (2002) conceptualized double loop learning as a method for leaders to reason in response to information. In defensive reasoning, staff members seek to avoid errors and suppress negative feelings about them, while productive reasoning leads staff to acknowledge errors and encourage open discussion about errors (Argyris, 1991). Argyris (1991) suggested that learning is beyond problem solving and more than mere motivation. Mohr (2005) highlighted the importance of leadership awareness of the active, double-loop learning style to affect safety results.

Hermeneutics: Hermeneutics and the hermeneutic circle align with the interpretative phenomenological methods of Heidegger. Patton (2002) noted the word hermeneutics derives from a Greek word meaning to understand or interpret. Shank (2006) stated hermeneutic research yields a shared understanding of issues.

Heuristic: Heuristic is a singular term to describe core cognitive strategies that ease workload (Sharps, Hess, Price-Sharps, & Teh, 2008). Smith (2005) defined heuristics as "hunches or rules of thumb" (p. 71).

Hierarchy: Hierarchy is a term that originally referred to clergy in a religious context (Walton, 2006). Walton defined hierarchy as "a group of individuals ranked according to authority, capacity, or position" (p. 229). Aron and Headrick (2002) noted the deep influence of health care's professional hierarchy to inhibit or transform culture change.

Interpretative Phenomenological Analysis (IPA): IPA is a qualitative research method and variation of phenomenology. Smith and Osborn (2008) suggested IPA involves a researcher exploring an insider's perspective of respondents to "make sense of their world" (p. 53). Larkin, Watts, and Clifton (2006) asserted the interpretative aspects of IPA, including participants' voices and contextual interpretation; researchers implementing IPA may "transcend or exceed the participants' own terminology and conceptualizations" (p. 113).

Interpretive Phenomenology: Conroy (2008) described interpretive phenomenology as a spiraling process similar to the hermeneutic circle. An element of historicity of the intended contextual framework combines with fore-structures of understanding in this Heideggerian philosophy (Conroy, 2008). The terms interpretative and interpretive are synonymous, signifying a manner of interpretation.

Lens: A lens is a theoretical qualitative research perspective with inductive examination of emerging themes during fieldwork (Creswell, 2003). The inductive examination includes a rich description of data, contexts, inferences, and conclusions (Cohen & Crabtree, 2008; Creswell, 2003; Trochim & Donnelly, 2008).

Medical error: Medical error is "failure of a planned action to be completed as intended or the use of a wrong plan to achieve an aim" (Kohn, Corrigan, & Donaldson, 1999). Baker, Day, & Salas (2006) noted medical errors resulting in loss of human life affect "families, staffs, communities, and health care providers' reputations" (p. 1588).

Patient safety: Patient safety is "freedom from accidental injuries stemming from the processes of health care" (Sutker, 2008, p. 9). Encinosa and Hellinger (2008) suggested barriers to patient safety occur at the systems level.

Phenomenology: Husserl described phenomenology as the essence of a matter or experience (Patton, 2002). Moustakas (1994) described phenomenology as an extensive study of a small number of respondents to generate understanding of patterns and meaning (Creswell, 2003). Although many variations of phenomenology are used in research, the two main philosophies are Husserlian (descriptive) and Heideggerian (interpretative) (van Manen, 2007). Heideggerian phenomenology aligns with hermeneutical underpinnings (Patton, 2002). Van Manen (2007) suggested the "practice of phenomenology" (p. 17) served to "mediate the epistemology of Husserl and ontology of Heidegger" (p. 18).

Privilege: Privilege is a concept of open information exchange between an investigator and a respondent while discussing an accident or incident with the sole purpose of safety improvements; policies, procedures, or laws protect information gathered during a privileged investigation from unauthorized disclosure (Patient Safety and Reporting Act, 2005; U.S. Air Force, 2007).

Root cause analysis: Root cause analysis is a process that originated from the systems safety community (Bahr, 1997;

Lu, Wetmore, & Przetak, 2006). This process includes drilling into underlying conditions of errors during investigation of adverse events (Bagian, 2005; Botwinick et al., 2006; Reason, 2000).

Safety culture: Silbey (2009) stated the earliest documented scholarly use of the term safety culture was in a 1986 report of the Chernobyl incident. Safety culture is a strategic philosophy implemented by leadership to enhance safety (Botwinick, Bisognano, & Haraden, 2006; Winokur & Beauregard, 2005). Leape et al. (2009) noted transparency as the "most important single attribute" (p. 425) to transform health care's safety culture.

Single loop learning: Argyris (2002) defined single loop learning as correcting errors without addressing the root causes. Holden (2009) suggested corrections that focus on blame or failure are ineffective to achieve organizational safety. Argyris (1991) described a doom loop as a single loop learning perspective where members (usually leaders) of an organization respond defensively or follow a course of action due to real or perceived management pressure.

Systems theory: Systems theory is acknowledgment of the ubiquity of error and the design and implementation of countermeasures and traps designed to counter human failings (Bahr, 1997; Reason, 2000; Senge, Kleiner, Roberts, Ross, & Smith, 1994).

Wrong-site surgery: Wrong-site surgery includes "surgical procedures performed on the wrong patient, wrong body part, wrong side of the body, or wrong level of a correctly-identified anatomic site" (Chodroff, 2007, p. 32). Holden (2009) suggested systems-based procedures to prevent wrong-site surgery are more effective than person-based corrections.

Index

A

Accountability, 152, 208, 300, 321, 326
Aha Moments, 73, 219, 220, 222-224, 230
Aeronautical Safety Centers, Military, 156
Apology, 286, 293-294
Authority Gradient, 165, 188-190
Autonomy, 66-67, 93, 192-193, 293-298, 302-303, 323, 334
Aviation Safety Reporting System, 207-209
Aviation Teamwork
  Contextual Framework, 72
  Methods, Heuristics, Ontology, 178
  Safety Methods, 64
Aviation Teamwork Heuristic, 72, 179
Aviation Teamwork Methods, 62-63, 76-88, 121, 125, 173-178
  Framework, 84
  Results in Health Care, 148, 186, 193-194
  Study Design, 96-100

B

Befindlichkeit, 69, 73-75, 154, 157, 178, 212, 215, 219, 222-228, 254, 260-261, 269-270, 287, 292, 318, 327-328, 337-338
Blame, 60-61, 132, 143, 147, 157, 168, 173, 203-205, 208, 210-211, 246-247, 260, 290, 293, 297, 323-325
Briefings, 159, 170, 201-205, 211

C

Central Research Questions, 82, 86-87, 107, 134
Checklist
    Aviation Origins, 159, 197-198
    Health Care Implementation, 198, 252, 267
Chernobyl, 140, 180
Cognition, 178
Communication, 61, 144-145, 150, 162, 166, 176, 183, 189-195, 201
    211, 238, 243-244, 262-264, 281, 297, 331
    Defined, 202
    Differences Between Physicians and Nurses, 203
    SBAR, 202
Confidentiality, 108, 112, 133, 207
Constructivist Perspective, Theory, 85, 105, 109-110, 218-222
Contextual Lens, 82, 118-121
Critical Theory, 217-219
Credibility, 100
    Equating in Qualitative Study, 109
Crew Resource Management
    Adaptation to Health Care, 141-142, 181-182, 190-196
    Air Florida Flight 90, 182-184
    As a Research Framework, 77-78, 99
    British Midlands 737, 188-189
    Components, 186
    Eastern 401, 162-163
    NASA Workshop, 81-82, 166
    Tenerife, 164
    Translating from Aviation to Health Care, 187-188, 237-238
    United 232, 185
    United Portland, OR Crash, 165

Culture
    Comparison of Aviation to Health Care Transformation, 66, 301
    Roots of Aviation Transformation, 61-62
    Teamworks culture, 64
Culture Transformation, 81-88

D

Decision Making, 190, 195, 335
Dependability, 118, 123-124, 128-129, 336
Disclosure, 125, 132-133, 144, 152, 273-274, 290, 292, 299, 300, 332
Double Loop Learning, 130-131, 179, 297, 302, 307, 323
    Defensive Reasoning, 130, 180
    Doom Loop, 180
    Pedagogy, conceptual foundation for theoretical framework, 181

E

Ego, 110, 246, 251--252, 295-296, 302-303, 330
Epistemology, 73-74
Error, 59-66
    Blameworthy Errors, 210
    Cognitive Errors, 186
    Medication Error, 142, 200-201, 239, 249, 277-279, 289
    Personal Struggle for Disclosure and Catharsis of Error Made, 291-292
    Research Question context, 87-88
    Root Causes, 76, 121-125, 140, 159, 177
Error Accounts, 276-286
Explication, 99, 111-120

F

Federal Aviation Administration, 77, 161, 166-168, 207, 304-305, 326, 332-333
Five Whys Theory, 147
Framework,
    Aviation to Health Care Context, 70, 81-84, 174-175
    Developing Study Research Questions, 77
    Health Care's Transformation Framework, 300, 309, 325, 328, 337
    Hermeneutical Framework Interpretation, 121
    Historicity and Basis for Interpretive Research, 212
    Researcher's Perspective — Aviation to Health Care, 213
    Teamwork Learning in Health Care, 245-246

G

Generational Differences, 309-314, 327, 334-335

H

Heidegger, 69, 73, 79, 121, 261, 298
Hermeneutic, 73, 79-82, 99, 111, 118, 120-121, 217, 222
Hermeneutic Circle, 81-82, 220, 254
    Point of Entry, 212
Hermeneutical Spiral, 218
Heuristic, 72, 178
Hierarchy, 66-67, 93, 144, 165-166, 297-298
    Health Care Training Philosophy, 322-323
Historicity, 70, 73, 81, 182, 212, 220
Husserl, 73

I

Implicit Learning, 217, 232, 245, 321
Interpretation, 82-84, 95, 108-111, 118-122, 128, 298-301, 307
    Provisional, 219-221
Interpretive Framework, 70, 125, 136, 212
Interpretive Phenomenology, 73, 79, 85, 97-99, 226, 254
    Double Hermeneutic, 120

J

Just Culture, 208

L

Leadership, 130, 142, 156, 176, 180, 184, 210, 233, 245, 269-276, 302, 307-308, 313, 317-318, 319, 322, 325-326, 330, 334-336
Leadership Philosophy, Author, 110
Learning Culture, 60, 70, 98, 130, 151-154, 230, 245, 297-299, 322-327
Limitations, 122-136, 295-296, 314

M

Mind-Mapping, 119, 226, 229
    Example, 128

N

National Transportation Safety Board, 77, 135, 182-184, 304, 326, 332-333

O

Ontology, 68, 73-75, 79, 93, 178, 212, 222, 302-303, 318, 327-328, 335
    Opportunity for Error Mitigation, 215
Organizational Culture, 68, 124-125, 140, 146, 186, 293, 324
Organizational Learning, 151, 191, 316

P

Pedagogy, 62, 181, 294, 299, 308, 330, 334-337
Phenomenology, 71-77, 80, 88, 217, 222
    Academic Rigor, 108-109
    Distillation Steps, 231
    Health Care Aspects Applied to Aviation, 336
    Heideggerian, 73
    Husserlian, 73
    Interpretive Phenomenology, Hermeneutical Underpinnings, 79, 85, 98, 216, 219
    Interpretative Phenomenological Analysis, 83-85
    Number of Study Participants, 105
    Study Purpose, 96
Physician Engagement, 190-192, 332
Pilots, 62, 65, 81, 161-165, 181-189, 197-198, 206, 296, 300-304, 325, 330-332
    Author Experience, 110, 199, 295
Pilot Study, 82, 107
Pilot Test, 127
Population (Study), 97, 100-105, 125, 129, 271
Privilege
    Military Safety Programs, 209
Productive Reasoning, 180-181
    Mindset, 130-131, 208-209, 242

Provisional Interpretation, 219
    Befindlichkeit, 219
Punishment, 63-64, 145, 208-210

Q

Qualitative Data, 76, 88, 121
Qualitative Methods, 71-76, 107-109, 119, 126, 129, 136, 196, 219, 328, 334

R

Real-Time Learning, 232, 241-245, 273, 299, 321
Researcher Identity, 121, 218-223
Researcher's Perspective, 83, 121
Root Cause, 76, 80, 96, 99, 121, 125, 137-140, 143-148, 151, 159, 162, 174, 201, 316, 328
    Health Care Education Foundations, 177, 293-294, 323
    Health Care Reporting Gaps, 201
Root Cause Analysis, 68, 110, 143, 211-212
    Challenger Disaster, 145, 302
Reporting, 78, 110, 140-143, 152-153, 159, 174-175, 205-211, 299-300, 315, 323
    Internal vs. External, 207, 211

S

Safety Culture, 68, 70, 98, 145, 151, 154, 192, 216, 337
    Aviation, 61, 72, 161-170, 173, 330-331
    Aviation to Health Care Researcher Comparison, 177, 223, 298, 301

Health Care Transformation, 58-59, 66, 76, 79-81, 88, 113, 122, 140-143, 148-149, 220-221, 230, 245, 293, 297, 299, 313, 321, 324, 327, 330, 337
Saturation, 105
Sense-Making, 69, 120, 123
Shared Understanding, 80, 125, 129, 295, 297, 336
Stratification, 100, 124-125
Structure, 116-117, 196, 246
Systems Safety, 143-144, 196

T

TeamSTEPPS, 196
Teamwork Ontology, 93, 178
Teamworks, 64, 173, 184-185, 187, 294, 296, 305-307, 316, 318, 321, 324-325, 337
    Core Values, 68, 224
    Goal, 296
    Vision, 68, 224
Tension, 66, 78, 221-223, 293, 322
Thematic Clustering, 108
Thematic Cluster(s), (ing), 114-118, 121, 231
Time Out, 202-203
To Err Is Human, 59, 63, 66, 254, 259
    Historicity Context, 182
Transcript(s), (ion), 99, 111-121, 128, 161-162, 229
Transferability, 129-130, 336
Transformation, 62-70, 78, 87, 93, 122, 179, 224-226, 254-260, 276, 290, 322, 329, 333
Transparency, 67, 111, 130, 135, 152, 173, 204, 209, 230, 260, 290, 293, 297, 299-303, 323, 332
Triangulation, 108-109

Trigger Phrases, 230, 233, 237
Two Challenge Rule, 203

W

Wright Brothers, 158-159, 172-173

References

Agency for Healthcare Research and Quality. (2009). *Hospital survey on patient safety culture: 2009 comparative database report* (AHRQ Publication No. 09-0030). Rockville, MD: Publisher.

Aggerwal, R., Undre, S., Moorthy, K., Vincent, C., & Darzi, A. (2004). The simulated operating theatre: Comprehensive training for surgical teams. *Quality and Safety in Health Care, 13,* i27-i32. doi: 10.1136/qshc.2004.010009

Airline Safety and Federal Aviation Administration Extension Act of 2010, 49 U.S.C. § 40101 (2010).

Alonso, A., Baker, D., Holtzman, A., Day, R., King, H., Toomey, L., & Salas, E. (2006). Reducing medical error in the military health system: How can team training help? *Human Resource Management Review, 16*(3), 396-415. doi: 10.1016/j.hrmr.2006.05.006

Argyris, C. (1991). Teaching smart people how to learn. *Harvard Business Review, 69*(3), 99-109. Retrieved from http://hbr.org/

Argyris, C. (2002). Double-loop learning, teaching, and research. *Academy of Management Learning and Education, 1*(2), 206-218. Retrieved from http://www.aom.pace.edu/amle/

Argyris, C. (2004). Reflection and beyond in research on organizational learning. *Management Learning, 35*(4), 507-509. doi: 10.1177/1350507604048276

Armitage, G. (2009). The risks of double checking. *Nursing Management, 16*(2), 30-35. Retrieved from http://journals.lww.com/nursingmanagment/pages/default/aspx

Aron, D., & Headrick, L. (2002). Educating physicians prepared to improve care and safety is no accident: It requires a systematic approach. *Quality and Safety in Healthcare, 11*(2), 168-173. doi: 10.1136/qhc.11.2.168

Bagian, J. (2005). Patient safety: What is really at issue? *Frontiers of Health Services Management 22*(1), 3-16.

Bahr, N. (1997). *System safety engineering and risk assessment: A practical approach.* New York: Taylor and Francis.

Baker, D., Day, R., & Salas, E. (2006). Teamwork as an essential component of high-reliability organizations. *Health Research and Educational Trust, 41*(4), 1576-1598. doi: 10.1111/j.1475-6773.2006.00566.x

Barlow, E. (2008). A simple checklist that saves lives. *Harvard Public Health Review*, Fall 2008.
Retrieved from www.hsph.harvard.edu

Bazerman, M. & Watkins, M. (2008). *Predictable surprises.* Boston: Harvard Business Press.

Berwick, D., & O'Kane, M. (2008). *National priorities and goals: Aligning our efforts to transform America's healthcare.* National Priorities Partnership. Washington, DC: National Quality Forum.
Retrieved from http://www.ahrq.gov

Besnard, D., Greathead, D., & Baxter, G. (2003). When mental models go wrong: co-occurrences in dynamic, critical systems. *International Journal of Human-Computer Studies, 60,* 117-128.
doi: 10.1016/j.ijhcs.2003.09.001

Beyea, S. (2007). Update on correct site surgery. *AORN Journal, 85*(2), 415-417.

Blendon, R., DesRochies C., & Brodie, M. (2002). Views of practicing physicians and the public on medical errors. *New England Journal of Medicine, 347,* 1933-1940.

Botwinick, L., Bisognano, M., & Haraden, C. (2006). *Leadership guide to patient safety.* Cambridge, MA: Institute for Healthcare Improvement. Retrieved from http://www.ihi.org

Bradbury-Jones, C., Irvine, F., & Sambrook, S. (2010). Phenomenology and participant feedback: Convention or contention? *Nurse Researcher, 17*(2), 25-33. Retrieved from http://nurseresearcher.rcnpublishing.co.uk/

Callendar, A., Hastings, D., Hemsley, M., Morris, L., & Peregrine, M. (2007, June). *Corporate responsibility and health care quality: A resource for health care boards of directors.* Retrieved from: http://www.ahrq.gov

Campbell, E., Regan, S., Gruen, R., Ferris, T., Rao, S., Cleary, P., & Blumenthal, D. (2007). Professionalism in medicine: Results of a national survey of physicians. *Annals of Internal Medicine, 147,* 795-802.

Carpenter, D. (2007). 'Never' land. *Hospitals & Health Networks, 81*(11), 34-38.
Retrieved from http://www.hhnmag.com/

Carroll, T., Gormley, T., Bilardo, V., Burton, R., & Woodman, K. (2006). Designing a new organization at NASA: An organizational design process using simulation. *Organization Science, 17*(2), 202-214.
doi: 10.1287/orsc.1050.0166

Catchpole, K., DeLeval, M., McEwan, A., Pigott, N., Elliott, M., McQuillan, A., ... Goldman, A. (2007). Patient handover from surgery to intensive care: using Formula 1 pit-stop and aviation models to improve safety and quality. *Pediatric anesthesia, 17,* 470-478. doi:10.1111/j.1460-9592.2007.02239.x

Chase, D., & McCarthy, D. (2010). Case study: Sustaining a culture of safety in the U.S. Department of Veterans Affairs health care system. Retrieved from http://www.commonwealthfund.org

Chodroff, C. (2007). Doing the "right" things to correct wrong-site surgery. *Patient Safety Authority, 4*(2), 29-45.

Clancy, C., & Tornberg, D. (2007). TeamSTEPPS: Assuring optimal teamwork in clinical settings. *American Journal of Medical Quality, 22*(3), 214-217. doi: 10.1177/1062860607300616

Clark, C. (2008). Student voices on faculty incivility in nursing education: A conceptual model. *Nursing Education Perspectives, 29*(5), 284-289.

Clarke, C. (2009). An introduction to interpretative phenomenological analysis: A useful approach for occupational therapy research. *British Journal of Occupational Therapy, 72*(1). 37-39. Retrieved from http://www.ingentaconnect.com/content/cot/bjot

Cohen, D., & Crabtree, B. (2008). Evaluative criteria for qualitative research in health care: Controversies and recommendations. *Annals of Family Medicine, 6*(4), 331-339. Retrieved from http://www.annfammed.org/

Colaizzi, P. (1978). Psychological research as the phenomenologist sees it. In R. S. Valle & M. King (Eds.), *Existential-phenomenological alternatives for psychology* (pp. 48-71). New York: Oxford University Press.

Conklin, T. (2007). Method or madness: Phenomenology as knowledge creator. *Journal of Management Inquiry, 16*(3), 275-287. doi: 10.1177/1056492607306023

Conway, J. (2005). Patient safety: The way we do the work. *Frontiers of Health Services Management, 22*(1), 45-49.

Conroy, S. (2008). A pathway for interpretive phenomenology. *International Journal of Qualitative Methods, 2*(3), 36-62. Retrieved from http://ejournals.library.ualberta.ca

Creswell, J. (2003). Research design: *Qualitative, quantitative, and mixed method approaches* (2nd ed.). Thousand Oaks, CA: Sage Publications.

Crowley, J., & Deen, J. (2009, May/June). Leadership practices to advance patient safety. *Patient Safety & Quality Healthcare,* May/June 2009 Vol. Retrieved from: www.psqh.com

Denham, C. (2007). TRUST: The 5 rights of the second victim. *Journal of Patient Safety, 3*(2), 107-119.

DeRosier, J., Stalhandske, E., Bagian, J., & Nudell, T. (2002). Using health care failure mode and effect analysis: The VA national center for patient safety's prospective risk analysis system. *The Joint Commission Journal, 27*(5), 248-267.
Retrieved from http://www.ahrq.gov

Downing, S. (2003). Validity: On the meaningful interpretation of assessment data. *Medical Education, 37*, 830-837.

Downing, T. (2010). Cometh the finest hour. *History Today, 60*(5), 25-29. Retrieved from Gale Academic Onefile website.

Dunn, E., Mills, P., Neily, J., Crittenden, M., Carmack, A., & Bagian, J. (2007). Medical team training: Applying crew resource management in the Veterans health administration. *The Joint Commission Journal on Quality and Patient Safety, 33*(6), 317-325.

Encinosa, W, & Hellinger, F. (2008). The impact of medical errors on ninety-day costs and outcomes: An examination of surgical patients. *Health Services Research, 43*(6), 2067-2085. doi: 10.1111/j.1475-6773.2008.00882.x

Espinoza, C., Ukleja, M., & Rusch, C. (2010). *Managing the millennials*. Hoboken, NJ: John Wiley & Sons.

Federal Aviation Administration. (2004). *AC120-51E crew resource management training*. Retrieved from http://www.faa.gov

Ferguson, J., & Fakelmann, R. (2005). The culture factor. *Frontiers of Health Services Management 22*(1), 33-40.

Fischer, M., Mazor, K., Baril, J. Alper, E., DeMarco, D., & Pugnaire, M. (2006). Learning from mistakes: Factors that influence how students and residents learn from medical errors. *Journal of General Internal Medicine, 21,* 419-423. Retrieved from Pub Med Central website.

Fleming, M., & Wentzell, N. (2008). Patient safety culture improvement tool: Development and guidelines for use. *Healthcare Quarterly, 11,* 10-15.

Flood, A. (2010). Understanding phenomenology. *Nurse Researcher, 17*(2), 7-15. Retrieved from http://nurseresearcher.rcnpublishing.co.uk/

Fosdick, G., & Uphoff, M. (2007). Adopting cross-industry best practices for measurable results. *Healthcare Executive, 22*(3), 14-20. Retrieved from http://www.ache.org

Gallagher, T., Waterman, A., Ebers, A., Fraser, V., & Levinson, W. (2003). Patients' and physicians' attitudes regarding the disclosure of medical errors. *JAMA, 289*(8), 1001-1007. Retrieved from http://www.jama.com

Garbutt, J., Waterman, A., Kapp, J., Dunagan, W., Levinson, W., Fraser, V., & Gallagher, T. (2008). Lost opportunities: How physicians communicate about medical errors. *Health Affairs, 27*(1), 246-255. Retrieved from http://www.healthaffairs.org

Gawande, A. (2007, December 10). The checklist. *The New Yorker.* Retrieved from http://www.newyorker.com/reporting/2007/12/10/071210fa_fact_gawande

Gawande, A. (2009). *The checklist manifesto.* New York: Metropolitan Books.

General Correspondence: Selfridge, Thomas E., 1907-1908, Wilbur and Orville Wright Papers, Manuscript Division, Library of Congress, Washington, D.C. Retrieved from http://www.loc.gov/

Giorgi, A. (2008). Concerning a serious misunderstanding of the essence of the phenomenological method in psychology. *Journal of Phenomenological Psychology, 39*(1), 33+. Retrieved from http://www.brill.nl/journal-phenomenological-psychology

Golafshani, N. (2003). Understanding reliability and validity in qualitative research. *The Qualitative Report, 8*(4), 597-607. Retrieved from http://www.nova.edu/ssss/ QR/QR8-4/golafshani.pdf

Groenewald, T. (2004). A phenomenological research design illustrated. *International Journal of Qualitative Methods, 3*(1), Article 4.
Retrieved from http://www.ualberta.ca/ ~iiqm/backissues/3_1/pdf/groenewald.pdf

Guise, J., Lowe, N., & Connell, L. (2008). Patient safety in obstetrics: What aviators, firefighters and others can teach us. *Nursing for Women's Health, 12*(3), 208-215. doi: 10.1111/j.1751-4865X.2008.00325.x

Hamman, W. (2004). The complexity of team training: What we have learned from aviation and its applications to medicine. *Quality and Safety in Health Care, 13*, i72-i79. doi: 10.1136/qshc.2004.009910

Haynes, A., Weiser, T., Berry, W., Lipsitz, S., Breizat, A., Dellinger, E., . . . Gawande, A. (2009). A surgical safety checklist to reduce morbidity and mortality in a global population. *New England Journal of Medicine, 360,* 491-499. doi: 10.1056/NEJMsa0810119

Healey, A., Undre, S., & Vincent, C. (2006). Defining the technical skills of teamwork in surgery. *Quality and Safety in Healthcare, 15,* 231-234.
doi: 10.1136/qshc.2005.017517

Heidegger, M. (1962). *Being and time.* New York: Harper and Row.

Helmreich, R. (1996). *The evolution of crew resource management.* Retrieved from http://www.psy.utexas.edu/psy/helmreich/iata96.htm

Helmreich, R., Merritt, A., & Wilhelm, J. (1999). The evolution of crew resource management training in commercial aviation. *International Journal of Aviation Psychology, 9*(1), 19-32.

Helmreich, R. (2000). On error management: Lessons from aviation. *BMJ, 320,* 781-785.

Helmreich, R., Musson, D., & Sexton, J. (2001). Applying aviation safety initiatives to medicine. *Focus on Patient Safety* 4(1), 1-2.

Helmreich, R., Wilhelm, J., Klinect, J., & Merritt, A. (2001). Culture, error, and crew resource management. In E. Salas, C. Bowers, & E. Edens (Eds.), *Improving teamwork in organizations* (pp. 302-331). Hillsdale, NJ: Erlbaum.

Horwitz, L., Krumholz, H., Green, M., & Huot, S. (2006). Transfers of patient care between house staff on internal medicine wards. *Archives of Internal Medicine, 166,* 1173-1177. Retrieved from http://www.archinternmed.com

Jablonski, E. (1982). *America in the air war.* Alexandria, VA: Time-Life.

Kalman, M., Wells, M., & Gavan, C. (2009). Returning to school: Experiences of female baccalaureate registered nurse students. *Journal of the New York State Nurses Association, 40*(1), 11-16.
Retrieved from http://www.nysna.org/publications/journal/journal.htm

Kaptchuk, T. (2003). Effect of interpretive bias on research evidence. *BMJ, 326,* 1453-1455.
Retrieved from http://www.bmj.com/

Kensella, E., Park, A., Applagyei, J., Chang, E., & Chow, D. (2008). Through the eyes of students: Ethical tensions in occupational therapy practice. *Canadian Journal of Occupational Therapy, 75*(3), 176-183. Retrieved from http://www.ingentaconnect.com/content/caot/cjot

Ketter, P. (2006). Soaring to new safety heights: Medical center changes workplace culture with innovative safety training program. *T + D, 60*(1), 51-54. Retrieved from http://www.astd.org/TD/

Kezar, A. (2000). The importance of pilot studies: Beginning the hermeneutic circle. *Research in Higher Education, 41*(3), 385-400.
Retrieved from http://www.springerlink.com/content/0361-0365/41/3/

Kliger, J., Blegen, M., Gootee, D., & O'Neil, E. (2009). Empowering frontline nurses: A structured intervention enables nurses to improve medication administration accuracy. *The Joint Commission Journal on Quality and Patient Safety, 35*(12), 604-612.

Kohn, L., Corrigan, J., & Donaldson, M. (1999). Committee on Quality of Health Care in America, Institute of Medicine: *To err is human: Building a safer health system.* Washington, DC: National Academy Press.

Kosnik, L., Brown, J., & Maund, T. (2007). Patient safety: Learning from the aviation industry. *Nursing Management, 38*(1), 25-30.
Retrieved from http://journals.lww.com/nursingmanagement/pages/default.aspx

Kottke, T., Solberg, L., Nelson, A., Belcher, D., Caplan, W., Green, L., . . . Woolf, S. (2008). Optimizing practice through research: A new perspective to solve an old problem. *Annals of Family Medicine, 6*(5), 459-462. doi: 10.1370/afm.862.

Kuzel, A., Woolf, S., Gilchrist, V., Engel, J., LaViest, T., Vincent, C., & Frankel, R. (2004). Patient reports of preventable problems and harms in primary health care. *Annals of Family Medicine, 2*(4), 333-340. Retrieved from http://www.annfammed.org/

Lancelot, J. (2007). Patient safety: Is technology enough? *Health Management Technology, 28*(12), 43-44. Retrieved from http://www.healthmgttech.com/

Larkin, M., Watts, S., & Clifton, E. (2006). Giving voice and making sense in interpretative phenomenological analysis. *Qualitative Research in Psychology, 3,* 102-120. doi: 10.1191/147808870qp062oa

Lazare, A. (2006). Apology in medical practice: An emerging clinical skill. *JAMA, 296*(11), 1401-1404. Retrieved from http://jama.ama-assn.org/

Leape, L., Berwick, D., Clancy, C., Conway, J., Gluck, P., Guest, J., . . . Isaac, T. (2009). Transforming healthcare: A safety imperative. *Quality and Safety in Health Care, 18,* 424-428. Retrieved from www.qshc.bmj.com

Leonard, M., Frankel, A., Simmonds, T., & Vega, K. (2004). *Achieving safe and reliable healthcare: Strategies and solutions.* Chicago: Health Administration Press.

Leonard, M., Graham, S, & Bonacum, D. (2004). The human factor: The critical importance of effective teamwork and communication in providing safe care. *Quality and Safety in Health Care, 13,* i85-i90. doi: 10.1136/qshc.2004.010033

Lessard, D. (2008). Assessing reduction of operating room team error using crew resource management principles. (Doctoral dissertation, Northcentral University, 2008). *Dissertation Abstracts International, 69, 11.*

Lewis, G., Vaithianathan, R., Hockey, P., Hirst, G., & Bagian, J. (2011). Counterheroism, common knowledge, and ergonomics: Concepts from aviation that could improve patient safety. *The Milbank Quarterly, 89*(1), 4-38.

Lewis, P., & Tully, M. (2009). Uncomfortable prescribing decisions in hospitals: The impact of teamwork. *Journal of the Royal Society of Medicine, 102,* 481-488. doi: 10.1258/jrsm.2009.090150

Looseley, A., Hotouras, A., Keogh, M. (2009). Patient safety and the aviation model: Medicine is still learning. *International Journal of Risk & Safety in Medicine, 21,* 131-137. doi: 10.3233/JRS-2009-0471

Lu, C-t., Wetmore, M., & Przetak, R. (2006). Another approach to enhance airline safety: Using management safety tools. *Journal of Air Transportation 11*(1), 113-139.
Retrieved from http://www.highbeam.com/publications/journal-of-air-transportation-p62290

Lyndon, A. (2008). Social and environmental conditions creating fluctuating agency for safety in two urban academic birth centers. *Journal of Obstetric, Gynecologic, and Neonatal Nursing, 37*(1), 13-23. doi: 10.1111/J.1552-6909.2007.00204.x

MacNulty, A., & Kennedy, D. (2008). Beyond the models: Investing in physician-hospital relationships. *Healthcare Financial Management, 62*(12), 72-77. Retrieved from http://www.hfma.org/Publications/hfm-Magazine/hfm-Magazine/

MacQueen, K., McLellan, E., Kay, K., & Milstein, B. (1998). Codebook development for team-based qualitative analysis. *Cultural Anthropology Methods, 10*(2), 31-36. Retrieved from http://www.cdc.gov/hiv/topics/surveillance/resources/software/pdf/codebook.pdf

Madden, T. (2005). *Cutting edge safety: Applying lean.* Retrieved from http://www.irmi.com

Mann, S., Marcus, R., & Sachs, B. (2006). Lessons from the cockpit: How team training can reduce errors on L&D. *Contemporary OB/GYN, 51*(1), 24-42.

Marshall, D., & Manus, D. (2007). A team training program using human factors to enhance patient safety. *AORN Journal, 86*(6), 994-1011.
Retrieved from http://www.aorn.org/AORNJournal/

Martin, J. (1993, November). Flying safety...We've come a long way. *Flying Safety*, 22-26.

Marx, D. (2001). *Patient safety and the "just culture": A primer for healthcare executives.* Prepared for Columbia University under a grant provided by the National Heart, Lung, and Blood Institute. Retrieved from California Hospital Patient Safety Organization website: www.chpso.org/lit/index.asp

McGreevy, J., Otten, T., Poggi, M., Robinson, C., Castaneda, D., & Wade, P. (2006). The challenge of changing roles and improving surgical care now: Crew resource management approach. *The American Surgeon, 72*(11), 1082-1087.
Retrieved from http://cms.sesc.org/opencms/opencms/as/index.html

Meyers, S. (2006). Standardizing safety. *Trustee, 59*(7), 12-14, 21. Retrieved from http://www.trusteemag.com/trusteemag_app/index.jsp

Mohr, J. (2005). Creating a safe learning organization. *Frontiers of Health Services Management, 22*(1), 41-44.

Morrow, S. (2005). Quality and trustworthiness in qualitative research in counseling psychology. *Journal of Counseling Psychology, 52*(2), 250-260.
doi: 10.1037/0022-0167.52.2.250

Moustakas, C. (1994). *Phenomenological research methods.* Thousand Oaks, CA: Sage.

Musson, D., & Helmreich, R. (2004). Team training and resource management in health care: Current issues and future directions. *Harvard Health Policy Review, 5*(1), 25-35.

National Transportation Safety Board. (1998a). *Factual report aviation: N651AA.*
Retrieved from http://www.ntsb.gov

National Transportation Safety Board. (1998b). *Report AAR-97/06.* Retrieved from http://www.ntsb.gov

National Transportation Safety Board. (2000). *Report AAR-00/03.* Retrieved from http://www.ntsb.gov

National Transportation Safety Board. (2003). *Factual report aviation: N963AS.*
Retrieved from http://www.ntsb.gov

National Transportation Safety Board. (2007). *Report AAR 07-01.* Retrieved from http://www.ntsb.gov/

National Transportation Safety Board. (2007). *Aviation accident statistics.*
Retrieved from http://www.ntsb.gov/aviation/Stats.htm

National Transportation Safety Board. (2009). *Speech at the National Press Club newsmaker luncheon*. Retrieved from http://www.ntsb.gov

National Transportation Safety Board. (2011). *Report AAR 11-02*. Retrieved from http://www.ntsb.gov/

Orlady, H. W. (1993). Airline pilot training today and tomorrow. In E. L. Weiner, B. G. Kanki, & R. L. Helmreich (Eds.), *Cockpit resource management* (pp. 451-453). San Diego: Academic Press, Inc.

Patient Safety and Quality Improvement Act, 42 U.S.C. § 299 (2005).

Patton, M. (2002). *Qualitative research & evaluation methods*, (3rd ed.). Thousand Oaks, CA: Sage.

Pawar, M. (2007, May). Getting beyond blame in your practice. *American Academy of Family Physicians*. Retrieved from http://www.aafp.org/fpm/20070500/30gett.pdf

Powell, S. (2007). Benefits to team briefings. *Healthcare Executive*, 22(4), 56-57.
Retrieved from http://www.ache.org/

Powell, S., & Hill, R. (2006). Home study program: My copilot is a nurse – using crew resource management in the OR. *AORN Journal*, 83(1), 178-206.
Retrieved from http://www.aorn.org/AORNJournal/

Pratt, S., Mann, S., Salisbury, M., Greenberg, P., Marcus, R., Stabile, B., . . . Sachs, B. (2007). Impact of CRM-based team training on obstetric outcomes and clinicians' patient safety attitudes. *The Joint Commission Journal on Quality and Patient Safety, 33*(12), 720-725.
Retrieved from: http://www:ahrq.gov

Pronovost, P., Weast, B., Holzmueller, C., Rosenstein, B., Kidwell, R., Haller, K., . . . Rubin, H. (2003). Evaluation of the culture of safety: Survey of clinicians and managers in an academic medical center. *Quality and Safety in Health Care, 12,* 405-410.
Retrieved from: www.qshc.bmj.com

Reason, J. (1997). *Managing the risks of organizational accidents.* Aldershot, England: Ashgate.

Reason, J. (2000). Human error: Models and management. *BMJ, 320,* 768-770.
Retrieved from http://www.bmj.com/

Roberts, R. (2007). The art of apology: When and how to seek forgiveness. *American Academy of Family Physicians.*
Retrieved from www.aafp.org/fpm

Rosen, A., Gaba, D., Meterko, M., Shokeen, P., Singer, S., Zhao, S., . . . Falwell, A. (2008). Recruitment of hospitals for a safety climate study: Facilitators and barriers. *The Joint Commission Journal on Quality and Patient Safety, 34*(5), 275-284.

Salas, E., Wilson, K., Burke, C., & Wightman, D. (2006). Does crew resource management training work? An update, an extension, and some critical needs. *Human Factors, 48*(2), 392-412.
Retrieved from http://www.hfes.org/

Salas, E., Almeida, S., Salisbury, M., King, H., Lazzara, E., Lyons, R., . . . McQuillan, R. (2009). What are the critical success factors for team training in health care? *The Joint Commission Journal on Quality and Patient Safety, 35*(8), 398-405.

Sax, H., Browne, P., Mayewski, R., Panzer, R., Hittner, K., Burke, R., & Coletta, S. (2009). Can aviation-based team training elicit sustainable behavioral change? *Archives of Surgery, 144*(12), 1133-1137.

Scannell-Desch, E., & Doherty, M. (2010). Experiences of U.S. military nurses in the Iraq and Afghanistan wars, 2003-2009. *Journal of Nursing Scholarship, 42*(1), 3-12. doi: 10:1111/j.1547-5069.2009.01329.x

Senge, P., Kleiner, A., Roberts, C., Ross, R., & Smith, B. (1994). *The fifth discipline fieldbook: Strategies and tools for building a learning organization.* New York: Doubleday.

Sexton, J., Thomas, E., & Helmreich, R. (2000). Error, stress, and teamwork in medicine and aviation: Cross sectional surveys. *BMJ, 320,* 745-749.

Shank, G. (2006). *Qualitative research: A personal skills approach* (2nd ed.). Upper Saddle River, NJ: Pearson Education, Inc.

Sharps, M., Hess, A., Price-Sharps, J., & Teh, J. (2008). Heuristic and algorithmic processing in English, mathematics, and science education. *The Journal of Psychology, 142*(1), 71-88.

Shojania, K., Fletcher, K., & Saint, S. (2006). Graduate medical education and patient safety: A busy – and occasionally hazardous – intersection. *Annals of Internal Medicine, 145*, 592-598. Retrieved from http://www.annals.org/

Small Deeds Count. (2007, February 18). *The Word for You Today*, p. 46.

Smedley, A. (2008). Becoming and being a preceptor: A phenomenological study. *Journal of Continuing Education in Nursing, 39*(4), 185-191. Retrieved from: http://www.ahrq.gov

Smerd, J. (2007). The silent treatment: 'Just be quiet about it.' *Workforce Management, 86*(20), 16-20. Retrieved from http://www.workforce.com/

Smith, J., & Osborn, M. (2008). Interpretative phenomenological analysis. In J. Smith (Ed.), *Qualitative psychology: A practical guide to research methods* (pp. 53-80). London: Sage.

Smith, M. (2005, January-February). Why did it take so long to make the diagnosis? *The Physician Executive*, January-February 2005, Vol. 70-72.

Smithsonian Institution, Presentation Ceremony, 17 December 1948, 1948-1949, Wilbur and Orville Wright Papers, Manuscript Division, Library of Congress, Washington, D.C.
Retrieved from http://www.loc.gov/

Spath, P., & Minogue, W. (2008). *The soil, not the seed: The real problem with root cause analysis.* Retrieved from Agency for Healthcare Research and Quality website: http://psnet.ahrq.gov

Stahel, P. (2008). Learning from aviation safety: A call for formal "readbacks" in surgery. *Patient Safety in Surgery, 2*(21), 1-2. doi: 10.1186/1754-9493-2-21

Stone, P., Harrison, M., Feldman, P., Linzer, M., Peng, T., Roblin, D., . . . Williams, E. (2005). Organizational climate of staff working conditions and safety – an integrative model. *Advances in Patient Safety from Research to Implementation.*
Retrieved from http://www.ahrq.gov/qual/advances/

Strauss, A., & Corbin, J. (1998). *Basics of qualitative research: Techniques and procedures for developing grounded theory.* Thousand Oaks, CA: Sage.

Sukkari, S., Sasich, L., Tuttle, D., Abu-Baker, A., & Howell, H. (2008). Development and evaluation of a required patient safety course. *American Journal of Pharmaceutical Education, 72*(3), 1-7.
Retrieved from http://www.ajpe.org/

Sutker, W. (2008). The physician's role in patient safety: What's in it for me? *Baylor University Medical Center Proceedings, 21*(1), 9-14.
Retrieved from http://www.baylorhealth.edu/Proceedings/

The Commonwealth Fund Commission on a High Performance Health System. (2008, July). *Why Not the Best? Results from the National Scorecard on U.S. Health System Performance.*
Retrieved from http://www.commonwealthfund.org

The Joint Commission. (2003, June 11). *Patient safety: Instilling hospitals with a culture of continuous improvement.* Testimony of D. O'Leary, M.D., President, Joint Commission before the Senate Committee on Governmental Affairs. Retrieved from http://www.jointcommission.org/NewsRoom/OnCapitolHill/testimony_061104.htm

The Joint Commission. (2006). *Applying aviation principles to health care: Crew resource management improves staff communication.*
Retrieved from http://www.jcipatientsafety.org

Thomas, E. (2006). *Aviation safety methods: Quickly adopted but questions remain.* Retrieved from Agency for Healthcare Research and Quality website: http://www.ahrq.gov

Thomas, S., & Pollio, H. (2004). *Listening to patients: A phenomenological approach to nursing research and practice.* New York: Springer Publishing Company.

Trochim, W., & Donnelly, J. (2008). *Research methods knowledge base* (3rd ed.). Mason, OH: South-Western.

United States Air Force. (2007). *Aircraft mishap investigations and the safety privilege.* Kirtland AFB, NM: Air Force Safety Center.

van Manen, M. (2007). Phenomenology of practice. *Phenomenology & Practice, 1*(1), 11-30. Retrieved from http://www.phandpr.org website

Wachter, R. (2010). Patient safety at ten: Unmistakable progress, troubling gaps. *Health Affairs, 29*(1), 1-9. doi: 10.1377/hithaff.2009.0785

Wall, C., Glenn, S., Mitchinson, S., & Poole, H. (2004). Using a reflective diary to develop bracketing skills during a phenomenological investigation. *Nurse Researcher, 11*(4), 20-29.
Retrieved from http://nurseresearcher.rcnpublishing.co.uk/

Walton, M. (2006). Hierarchies: The Berlin Wall of patient safety. *Quality & Safety in Health Care, 15*(4), 225-226. Retrieved from http://qualitysafety.bmj.com

Weiner, E., Kanki, B., & Helmreich, R. (1993). *Cockpit resource management.* San Diego: Academic Press, Inc.

Weiner, E., & Nagel, D. (1988). *Human factors in aviation.* San Diego: Academic Press, Inc.

Wells, A., & Rodrigues, C., (2004). *Commercial aviation safety* (4th ed.). New York: McGraw Hill.

Wells, L. (2007). Role of Information Technology in Evidence Based Medicine: Advantages and Limitations. *Internet Journal Of Healthcare Administration, 4*(2), 5.

Williams, L. (2008). The value of a root cause analysis. *Long-Term Living: For the Continuing Care Professional, 57*(11), 34-37. Retrieved from www.ltlmagazine.com/

Winokur, S., & Beauregard, K. (2005). Patient safety: Mindful, meaningful, and fulfilling. *Frontiers of Health Services Management, 22*(1), 17-28.

Wong, R., Saber, S., Ma, I., & Roberts, J. (2009). Using television shows to teach communication skills in internal medicine residency. *BMC Medical Education, 9*(9), 1-8. doi: 10.1186/1472-6920-9-9

Wood, R. (2003). *Aviation safety programs: A management handbook* (3rd ed.). Englewood, CO: Jeppesen-Sandersen.

Yin, R. (2003). *Case study research* (3rd ed.). Thousand Oaks, CA. Sage.

Zikmund, W. (2003). *Business research methods* (3rd ed.). Mason, OH: South-Western.

Appendix A

Phenomenological Interview Guide

Learning

- What has been your experience with learning aviation teamwork methods?

- Could you go back to your first thoughts when you began to learn about aviation teamwork methods in a health care context?
    - Describe your initial judgments of these practices.
    - What made sense? What was confusing?
    - How did you learn? From culture or background; anecdotal vs. science perspective? Was it from a coherent curriculum or ad hoc?

- o Do you have any vivid memories of this experience?

- How would you describe learning in the context of the organizational and departmental climate where you work?

- With what tasks and in which contexts are aviation teamwork methods *most critical* to **learn** in your area of responsibility?
    - o Crew resource management (CRM)
    - o Briefings
    - o Checklists
    - o Reporting and analyzing
    - o Another area?

- What is your experience with learning how to respond to errors on the job made by yourself or someone else? When you first learned about responding to errors, how did you feel?

- Describe your experience with learning to use technology or other programs or initiatives to transform the safety culture of your department or organization.

Application

- How do you describe your experience applying aviation teamwork methods in health care settings to mitigate root causes of medical errors?

- Could you go back to your first experiences of applying aviation teamwork methods in a health care context?
    - Describe your initial successes or failures.
    - Was the experience with yourself only or with others?
    - Did you discuss the experience with others or comment on it?
    - Do you have any vivid memories of your experience?

- With what tasks and in which contexts are aviation teamwork methods *most critical* to **apply** in your area of responsibility?
    - Crew resource management (CRM)?
    - Briefings?
    - Checklists?
    - Reporting and analyzing?
    - Another area?

- Looking back upon your experience of learning to respond to errors, how would you describe how this experience transformed your work over time? How have you applied this experience?

- Describe an experience of a health care provider recovering from making an error and going through grief, anxiety, healing, and so forth.
    - Are apologies—acknowledgement, explanation, remorse, reparation—part of organizational strategies?

- Describe any situations where you are aware that aviation teamwork methods are misapplied or underutilized. Other thoughts?

Conclusion

- As we conclude the discussion, what stands out as an important theme or experience?

- Did you learn anything new based on this discussion?

- Please provide any other observations you may have regarding aviation teamwork methods in health care, or anything else you consider important regarding the research problem, purpose, or questions.

Appendix B

Respondent Recruiting Letter

Dear Health Care Colleague:

My name is Mitchell Morrison, and I am a Doctor of Philosophy (Ph.D.) candidate in the School of Business and Technology Management at Northcentral University (NCU). In my dissertation research, I am pursuing a qualitative study using phenomenology to explore, describe, and interpret learning and application of aviation teamwork methods in health care settings to mitigate medical errors.

As a Ph.D. researcher, I am seeking to interview a purposively selected group of respondents from Northern California health care organizations, including physicians, nurses, anesthesiologists, residents, and patient safety managers. To qualify for the study, respondents must be willing to discuss their experience with aviation teamwork methods applied in health care settings to mitigate medical errors. For purposes of the study, aviation teamwork methods include Crew Resource Management (CRM), checklists, briefings, and reporting-investigating. Research will take place during scheduled 60-90 minute semi-structured, one-on-one, audio-taped interviews at a quiet, pre-determined private location. Interviews will be transcribed verbatim, and after initial analysis I will provide a debriefing (in person or telephone) to mutually confirm emergent themes and enhance the study's credibility.

I will strictly adhere to HHS research protocols. I have received NCU Institutional Review Board (IRB) approval to begin research and plan to complete required approval processes to conduct research within your organization. I will provide a clear explanation of study goals and potential outcomes to potential respondents and will answer any questions regarding the study. Prior to data collection, I will provide a written informed consent agreement to be signed by both parties.

NCU is an accredited university specializing in exclusively online degree programs. I am an active-duty Coast Guard aviator with 28 years' service, Airline Transport Pilot-rated, with 6,600 flying hours in airplanes and helicopters. I hold the rank of Commander and serve as the Executive Officer (second in command) of Air Station Sacramento at McClellan Field. I am also an Embry-Riddle Aeronautical University adjunct faculty member and have taught various graduate/undergraduate aeronautical science and aviation safety courses. I reside in Sacramento's North Natomas community.

Please contact me if you or a colleague desire to participate in the study.

Warm regards,
Mitchell Morrison

Appendix C

Informed Consent Form

Understanding Health Care's Safety Culture Transformation:
A Phenomenological Study of Error Mitigation through Aviation Teamwork

Purpose

You are invited to participate in a research study being conducted for a dissertation at Northcentral University in Prescott Valley, Arizona. The purpose of this qualitative study is to use phenomenology to explore, describe, and interpret health care respondent experiences with aviation teamwork methods to mitigate root causes of medical errors. The phenomenon to explore will be learning and application of aviation teamwork methods in health care settings to mitigate root causes of medical errors.

There is no deception in this study. We are interested in your opinions and reflections about health care's safety culture transformation.

Participation Requirements

A short telephone interview will serve as a screening tool for further purposive selection from Northern California health care organizations for a private 60-90 minute audio-taped interview.

Research Personnel

The following people are involved in this research project and may be contacted at any time: *Mitchell Morrison, Ph.D. Candidate, (xxx) xxx-xxxx, (home); (xxx) xxx-xxxx (cell). Dr. Steve Roussas, Supervising Dissertation Chair, (xxx) xxx-xxxx.* Note: phone numbers redacted post-study for privacy.

Potential Risk/Discomfort

Although there are no known risks in this study, some of the information is personally sensitive and also includes questions about medical errors, which may be distressing to some people. However, you may withdraw at any time and you may choose <u>not</u> to answer any question that you feel uncomfortable in answering.

Potential Benefit

There are no direct benefits to you of participating in this research. No incentives are offered. Additional research will benefit clinical outcomes regarding the impacts of aviation methods.

Anonymity/Confidentiality

The data collected in this study are confidential. All data are coded such that your name is not associated with them. In addition, the coded data are made available only to the researchers associated with this project. Pseudonyms will be used in quotes or in descriptive narratives.

Right to Withdraw

You have the right to withdraw from the study at any time without penalty. You may decline to answer interview questions if you do not want to answer them.

We would be happy to answer any question that may arise about the study. Please direct your questions or comments to: *Mitchell Morrison, Ph.D. Candidate, (xxx) xxx-xxxx (home); (xxx) xxx-xxxx (cell).*

Signatures

I have read the above description of: Understanding Health Care's Safety Culture Transformation: A Phenomenological Study of Error Mitigation through Aviation Teamwork study and understand the conditions of my participation. My signature indicates that I agree to participate in the experiment.

Participant's Name: _____

Researcher's Name: _____

Participant's Signature: _____

Researcher's Signature: _____

Date: _____

Appendix D

Schematics

Figure D1. Data Collection

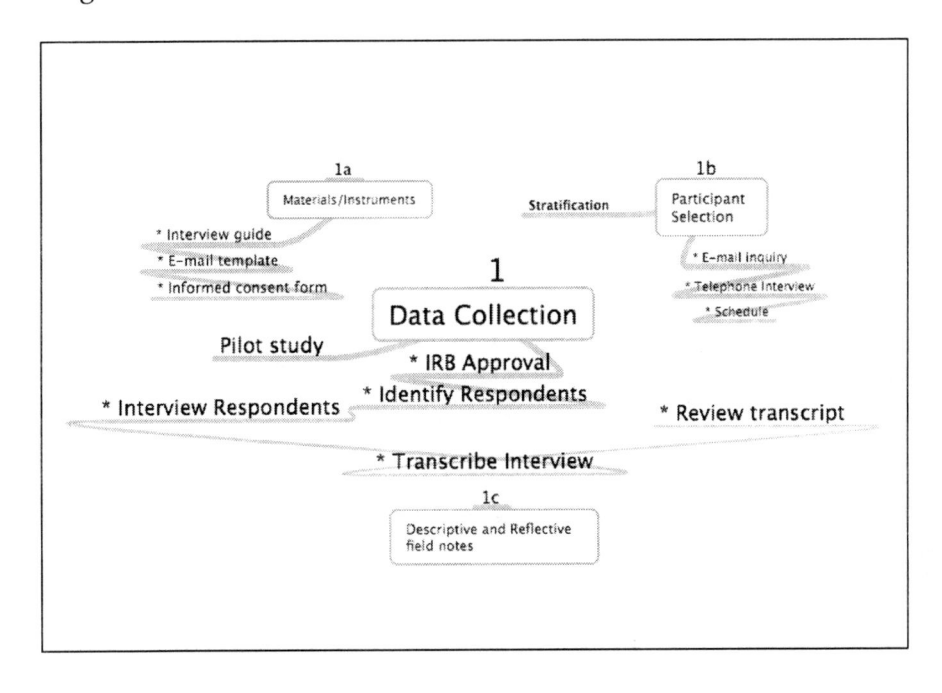

Figure D2. Exploration

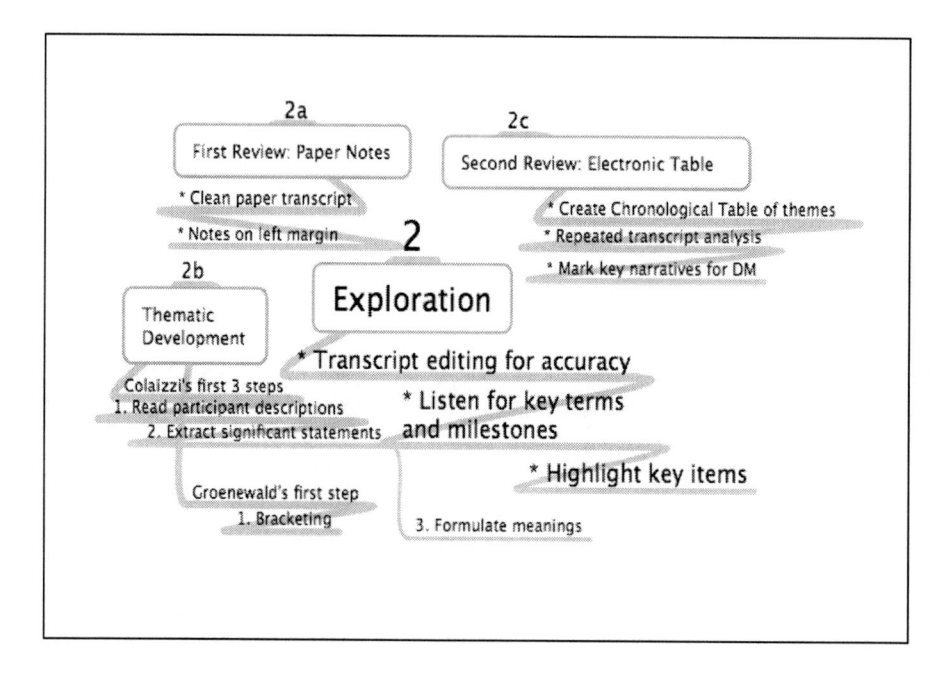

2a First Review: Paper Notes
* Clean paper transcript
* Notes on left margin

2c Second Review: Electronic Table
* Create Chronological Table of themes
* Repeated transcript analysis
* Mark key narratives for DM

2 Exploration

2b Thematic Development

Colaizzi's first 3 steps
1. Read participant descriptions
2. Extract significant statements

Groenewald's first step
1. Bracketing

* Transcript editing for accuracy
* Listen for key terms and milestones
* Highlight key items

3. Formulate meanings

Figure D3. Descriptive Analysis

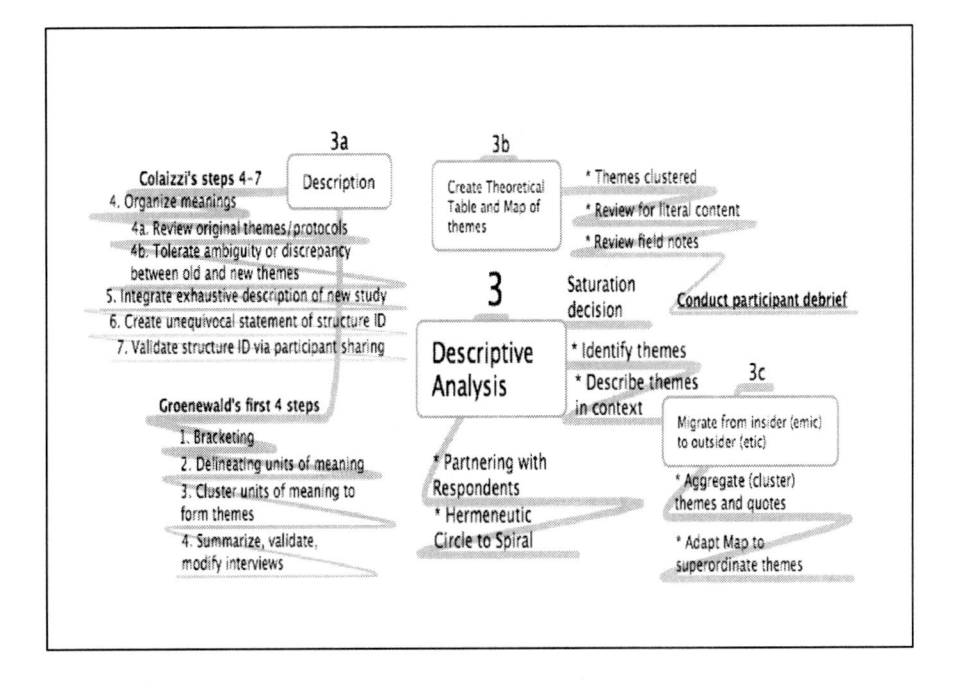

	3a	3b	
Colaizzi's steps 4–7	Description	Create Theoretical Table and Map of themes	* Themes clustered * Review for literal content * Review field notes
4. Organize meanings			
4a. Review original themes/protocols			
4b. Tolerate ambiguity or discrepancy between old and new themes			
5. Integrate exhaustive description of new study			
6. Create unequivocal statement of structure ID			
7. Validate structure ID via participant sharing			

3 Descriptive Analysis

Saturation decision — Conduct participant debrief

* Identify themes
* Describe themes in context

Groenewald's first 4 steps
1. Bracketing
2. Delineating units of meaning
3. Cluster units of meaning to form themes
4. Summarize, validate, modify interviews

* Partnering with Respondents
* Hermeneutic Circle to Spiral

3c
Migrate from insider (emic) to outsider (etic)

* Aggregate (cluster) themes and quotes
* Adapt Map to superordinate themes

Figure D4. Interpretive Analysis

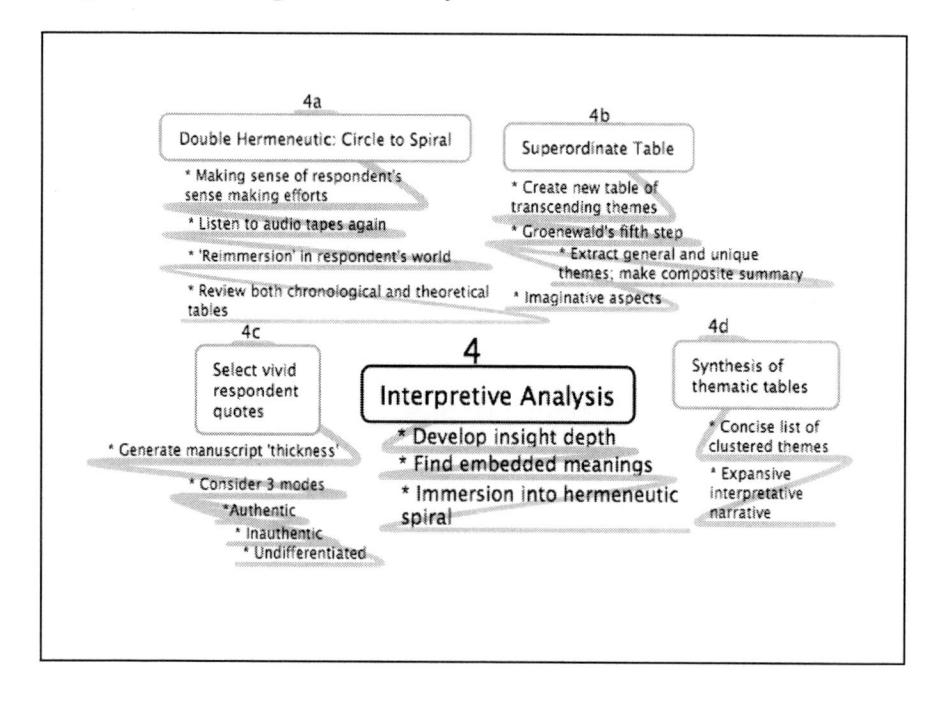

4a Double Hermeneutic: Circle to Spiral
* Making sense of respondent's sense making efforts
* Listen to audio tapes again
* 'Reimmersion' in respondent's world
* Review both chronological and theoretical tables

4b Superordinate Table
* Create new table of transcending themes
* Groenewald's fifth step
* Extract general and unique themes; make composite summary
* Imaginative aspects

4c Select vivid respondent quotes
* Generate manuscript 'thickness'
* Consider 3 modes
  *Authentic
  * Inauthentic
  * Undifferentiated

4 Interpretive Analysis
* Develop insight depth
* Find embedded meanings
* Immersion into hermeneutic spiral

4d Synthesis of thematic tables
* Concise list of clustered themes
* Expansive interpretative narrative

works

www.wxrks.com

CPSIA information can be obtained at www.ICGtesting.com
Printed in the USA
BVOW081513200613

323820BV00002B/4/P